Praise for Feminine Genius

"LiYana Silver could be writing about anything—from mushroom collecting to the stock market—and my heart would sing. Her writing is gorgeous, and this praise comes from a passionate lover of language. But it happens that LiYana Silver is writing about the blazing heart of the human experience. Her description of and loving guidance into the fruitful darkness is among the very wisest and most lyrical I have encountered. I will return to that section again and again. This book unraveled and rewove the fabric of my femininity, and hence my humanity. Deep bow."

MIRABAI STARR
author of *Caravan of No Despair: A Memoir of Loss and Transformation* and *Teresa of Avila: Passionate Mystic*

"LiYana's book is a powerful invitation for women to step into their biggest, brightest, truest, most powerful selves. I was truly blown away by the wisdom and inspiration on each page. If you're a woman ready to embrace her feminine power, this book is a must read."

ALEXANDRA JAMIESON
functional nutrition coach, co-creator of *Super Size Me*, and author of *Women, Food, and Desire: Embrace Your Cravings, Make Peace with Food, Reclaim Your Body*

"LiYana Silver's *Feminine Genius* is a courageous, wise, juicy book that redefines the genre of women's empowerment. This timely work is a lively love letter to women to tap into their feminine brilliance. With a fresh, readable style, Silver guides us with stories, practices, and heartfelt insights that are meaningful and potent. This bold book asks women to step into their special birthright, and it provides just the right mix of spirituality, smarts, and sassiness to get the job done. Brava. Highly recommended!"

MARC DAVID
author of *The Slow Down Diet: Eating for Pleasure, Energy, and Weight Loss* and *Nourishing Wisdom: A Mind-Body Approach to Nutrition and Well-Being;* founder of Institute for the Psychology of Eating

"LiYana Silver's brand-new book lofts her and her readers right up to the stratosphere of feminine genius that she so accurately describes. It's impossible to dive into these pages without coming out restored, refreshed, renewed, and connected to a power that has always been each of ours to own. *Feminine Genius* is a down-to-earth, deeply useful guide; a must-read for every woman!"

REGENA THOMASHAUER
New York Times bestselling author of *Pussy: A Reclamation*
and founder of Mama Gena's School of Womanly Arts (mamagenas.com)

"This book is exactly what women need to remember who we are and how to access our unique genius. And this unique brand of genius is exactly what the world needs right now, too. This book is brilliant and right on time."

KATE NORTHRUP
bestselling author of *Money: A Love Story*

"This book is a must for anyone (men, too) on a path to wake up, be fully human, and find the magic of being fully alive. LiYana offers a clear path—with joy, pleasure, and juiciness—to remembering the Divine Feminine in all of us. She offers us stories, exercises, humor, and a bright shiny mirror into the depths of our feminine souls aching to be seen and loved. What a loving gift LiYana has given us in this radical, articulate, wise, and boldly true practice of cultivating our Feminine Genius. I know that as more of us embrace the deep wisdom in this book, the more our species will heal and the more our culture will be in balance."

MARY WALDNER, LMFT
cofounder and Chief Consciousness Officer at Mary's Gone Crackers®

"For any woman doubting herself, her body, her value, her potential, her sexuality, or her femininity, *Feminine Genius* is a needed re-education and a bold proclamation. If you wish to lead a more boundless, joyful life, I wish this book for you."

AMANDA STEINBERG
founder of DailyWorth and author of *Worth It*

"*Feminine Genius* is one of the most potent books I've ever read. LiYana Silver is a master of metaphor and teaches women the lessons we critically need to learn to feel healthy and whole in an unforgettable, soul-wrenching way. Her writing is a soothing and energizing antidote to the toxic conditioning of our patriarchal culture. All I wanted to do was stay home and read it from cover to cover! I recommend every woman do the same."

JENA LA FLAMME
author of *Pleasurable Weight Loss: The Secrets to Feeling Great,
Losing Weight,* and *Loving Your Life Today* (jenalaflamme.com)

"*Feminine Genius* is a wake-up call for women. It touches upon our deepest places of shame and hope—our bodies, feelings, sexuality, intuition, spirituality, and womanhood—and shows us how what we thought were our greatest liabilities are actually some of our greatest strengths.

We as women still need help to feel less crazy as we walk the path of the messiness and the magic of life. *Feminine Genius* gives us useful tools to change what is no longer working. It also shows us how to give up the Inner Mean Girl crazy-making of constant self-improvement and simply become truly happy and fully ourselves right now.

Devour its pages and feel yourself shine brighter. And then, as quickly as you can, introduce this book to all the women you love."

AMY AHLERS
founder of Mama Truth Circle, author of *Big Fat Lies Women
Tell Themselves,* and coauthor of *Reform Your Inner Mean Girl*

"What LiYana has created here is a path back to your feminine identity. Reading each chapter, you will be able to name and claim a piece of yourself that may have gotten lost in masculine culture. Doing this process will put you back in your body so you can navigate through your life with your voice, your soul, your desire, and your joy as your compass. An important spiritual feminist read."

ALISA VITTI
author of *WomanCode: Perfect Your Cycle, Amplify Your Fertility, Supercharge
Your Sex Drive, and Become a Power Source* and founder of FLOliving.com

"With delicious candor and well-earned womanly wisdom, LiYana Silver will guide you home to your *Feminine Genius*. Like a sage and sassy girlfriend, she'll help you navigate both the darkest and the brightest corners of your inner landscape. If you're wondering how to embrace the unique twists and turns of your own initiation into Womanhood, Feminine Genius offers invaluable support."

SARA AVANT STOVER
author of *The Way of the Happy Woman* and *The Book of SHE:
Your Heroine's Journey into the Heart of Feminine Power*

"For several thousand years, the world has rewarded masculine ways of being and punished feminine ways. But that world is changing rapidly; the patriarchy is in its end times. LiYana Silver's new book shows the way forward to a future in which feminine wisdom is appreciated, respected, and rewarded just as much as masculine wisdom. *Feminine Genius* is an important roadmap towards success in a post-patriarchal world."

MICHAEL ELLSBERG
author of *The Education of Millionaires*
and coauthor of *The Last Safe Investment*

"LiYana Silver's words are not just another theory or rote neo-goddess dogma. *Feminine Genius* is a living, authentic, embodied oracle for any woman who truly desires to live her fullest, most sovereign self."

DR. SAIDA DÉSILETS
women's empowerment coach and author of
Emergence of the Sensual Woman (SaidaDesilets.com)

"Articulate, insightful, and compassionate, LiYana's deep feminine wisdom will illuminate your path to living a turned-on life. She's a wise guide who will inspire and encourage you to discover your own Feminine Genius."

SHERI WINSTON
Wholistic Sexuality™ teacher and author of *Women's Anatomy
of Arousal and Succulent SexCraft* (IntimateArtsCenter.com)

"*Feminine Genius* is a delectable treat with an extra helping of smart sauce in a flambé of raw truth. It delivers the deep nourishment our collective feminine spirit is so hungry for. It's been my privilege to see firsthand how LiYana walks her talk with the utmost integrity. This book is a reflection of her capacity to shine that light—vibrating with Shakti, sensuality, unflinching honesty, and fierce love."

LISA SCHRADER
women's sacred sensuality coach, author of *Kama Sutra 52:
A Year's Worth of the Best Positions for Passion and Pleasure,*
and founder of AwakeningShakti.com

"Read the book *Feminine Genius* and you'll discover that LiYana Silver has been quietly living the all-too-common and frequently painful experience of woman so she could write the words we each need to hear and lay down the truth with such elegance and artistry that all who read it will blossom into the women we are longing to become. It's rare to say about a 'self-help' style book, but it's truly breathtaking."

ALEXIS NEELY
family wealth lawyer, mom, and founder of
New Law Business Model & Eyes Wide Open Life

"From shadow to light, LiYana navigates the complexity of modern, patriarchal life to make room for the Sacred Feminine in us all—a genius the world cannot survive without. Jump on this train and let the spiral begin!"

CHANTAL PIERRAT
founder of Emerging Women

Feminine Genius

Feminine Genius

The Provocative Path to
Waking Up and Turning On
the Wisdom of Being a Woman

LIYANA SILVER

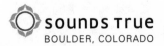

sounds true
BOULDER, COLORADO

Sounds True
Boulder, CO 80306

© 2017 LiYana Silver

Published 2017

Cover design by Rachael Murray
Book design by Beth Skelley

Printed in Canada

Library of Congress Cataloging-in-Publication Data
Names: Silver, LiYana, author
Title: Feminine genius : the provocative path to waking up
   and turning on the wisdom of being a woman / LiYana Silver.
Description: Boulder, CO : Sounds True, 2017.
Identifiers: LCCN 2016048508 (print) | LCCN 2017002839 (ebook) |
   ISBN 9781622038299 (pbk.) | ISBN 1622038290 (pbk.) |
   ISBN 9781622038305 (ebook) | ISBN 1622038304 (ebook)
Subjects: LCSH: Women—Psychology. | Self.
Classification: LCC HQ1206 .S525 2017 (print) | LCC HQ1206 (ebook) |
   DDC 305.42—dc23
LC record available at https://lccn.loc.gov/2016048508

10 9 8 7 6 5 4 3 2 1

To you

To every woman from whose torch
I light my own: Even if I do not know you,
still I bow to you.

And to you, woman,
reading this right now: As says the poet Rumi,
"You suppose you are the trouble, but you are the cure."

Contents

Part One

Going to the Source

1

You Are Not Crazy
The World Is Off Its Rocker

When you are at war with yourself and you win,
who loses?
CARL BUCHHEIT

The world has gone stark raving, totally loony tunes, round the bend, nutty as a fruitcake, not in its right mind, dangerously and absolutely mad. And you can't see all the ways the world is wacky because you marinate in them—you literally stew in them—day in and day out. And you not only swim in the stuff, you drink it for breakfast, lunch, and dinner, so the insanity becomes part of your bones, your blood, and your DNA.

It is as though you—like most women—walk around in a straight jacket and a muzzle, and you've been wearing them so long, and they feel so normal, that you no longer even notice that you are bound, gagged, and hobbled. Instead, you gaze in the mirror, examine your reflection, and ask, "How do I look? Do these handcuffs make me look fat?"

This, my friend, is crazypants.

In my decade and a half as a coach, seeing this all day, every day, one hundred times over and in a thousand variations (not to mention within my own self), has confirmed for me that both the world out there and the world within far too many women need a big, bold do-over. A new era, inspired from our sorely missed, pro-goddess past and informed by each woman's true wisdom, must become our new normal. And you, sister, like me and like every woman, bring your piece of the magic so that together we can make our worlds over.

And yet, as one of my mentors, Carl Buchheit, asks, "When you are at war with yourself and you win, who loses?"

Oh, right. That war inside you. There's that.

Let me share with you how I came to be writing these words, and why I believe that cultivating Feminine Genius is the key to bringing an end to the war we each wage against ourselves—and perhaps even to the war that the world at large wages against women.

My own path to an inner cease-fire began on the stage—well, actually on the side of the stage, cozied up in my pint-sized sleeping bag while my mother led her dance rehearsals. Aside from a brief time when I wanted to be a princess, and then a scientist, I had always wanted to become a professional dancer like my mom was. When my father, a staunch proponent of following your bliss, asked me why I loved to dance so much, I told him, "Daddy, I feel like I have this light inside of me, and when I dance people get to see it too. I just want to share it."

So when I turned sixteen, I got myself a scholarship and left my hippie home in northern New Mexico to go to a fancy boarding school for the arts in conservative New England. I quickly memorized the script I would need to follow if I were to go pro: be very, very thin and get the steps very, very right. These harsh rules apply for a girl aspiring to be a dancer as well as for a girl aspiring to be a woman. On both accounts, I got busy. I shifted my focus from sharing my light to getting it right, from following my bliss to following the script, and from shakin' my booty to working my ass off.

Along with biology, French, and ballet classes, I studied up on how to become an excellent anorexic, and embraced my new way of life with religious fervor. I ate nearly nothing. I scrutinized the girls who were technically advanced and tried not only to dance like them, but also to move like them, sit like them, and even talk like them. I stayed late in the dance studios, practicing long past the point of pain and fatigue. As the weeks and months went on, people asked with concern if I was getting too thin, but I knew other students were secretly jealous of me and my teachers were proud of me.

During one visit home, I handed my parents my report card—a column of straight As—and waited for their reaction. Instead of admiring the piece of paper, they looked at me and beamed. "You know," my father said, "we love you unconditionally. Always will. There is nothing you could do or not do to change that."

While that was probably the best thing any girl could hope to hear from the god and goddess of her universe, inside I was distraught. *No, I thought. No! Don't you understand? I don't deserve that. Not yet. There are so many things wrong with me, so many ways I am not yet perfect. I can't accept your love until then.*

Back in boarding school, I was hungry, tired, and felt like I was holding my breath all the time. I dreamt at night about the indulgences I wouldn't let myself have by day, things like meat with gravy, ice cream sundaes, boys to kiss. I longed to skip class and sleep in. I started to feel that the urges of my body—my hungry, unruly, feminine body—were antithetical to my goals of becoming a great dancer. I began to believe that somehow my body was against me.

I doubled down with my preferred war tactics of control and deprivation, and didn't look up for the next ten years. One day, in my twenties, in rehearsal for a dance company I dearly loved, I watched a fellow dancer practice. As I stretched on the side of the room, an icy realization poured into my body. She was a great technician (she got the steps very, very right), yet as I watched her, I became aware that her greatness was about something far beyond her technical virtuosity. She seemed completely at home in herself. A luminescence shone from her that was almost holy. In that third-story dance studio in Lower Manhattan, it hit me in the gut: I would never feel truly successful, in dance or otherwise, because I was focused too much on following my script and too little on sharing my light.

But the light I saw in my fellow dancer woke up a dormant part of me. I realized that I gravely missed my light, even if I had no idea how to regain it. I realized that I had traveled far from my true self, and the path back was anything but clear. Regardless, more than the salvation that I thought my script would offer me and that I was killing myself to reach, I began instead to want to feel completely at home in myself. I longed to feel luminous and to know myself as holy—or, if that was too much to ask, then to just feel okay.

Although I didn't know it at the time, it was my *want* that was actually my first step on the path that led back to me. It was my *longing* that let me pick up that humble white flag that signifies the end of a war. Friend, I believe you picked up this book because you also feel a similar *longing* stirring in you.

Maybe you too, at some time in your girlhood, were naturally in touch with your light. Maybe you too, like the women I get to know and get to work with, used to feel naturally confident in your body, sassy (in my case also bossy), and clear about what you wanted. Even if you have to reach way, way, way back into your past, you might find a time when pleasure was everywhere for you, as natural as drawing breath. When you were luminescent. When you felt what you felt, knew what you knew, and you felt completely at home in yourself.

And then maybe at some point either very early on or in young womanhood, your light began to dim, or the world dimmed it for you. It became no longer safe to feel what you felt and to know what you knew. Your body might have even stopped feeling like your own and became a commodity to trade for love, acceptance, and belonging—if only you could become "perfect." You learned to hold your tongue, be a good girl, close your legs, and do as you were told. Your girlhood was cut short. You stopped trusting yourself. You stopped hearing your soul.

GOING MAD

To give you a bigger, clearer picture of how insane things truly are, and how the insanity at large skews a woman's everyday reality, allow me to present to you a few facts and figures. Fasten your seatbelts, because it's a bit of a nauseating ride. Although women make up 51 percent of the population, we hold only about 11 percent of decision-making and policy-setting positions in media, government, and education.[1]

Eighty-one percent of ten-year-olds worry about becoming too fat.[2] A woman is 70 percent more likely than a man to experience depression during her lifetime.[3] One in four women takes antidepressants, and women use antianxiety medications at almost twice the rate of men.[4] Sixty-five percent of American women have an eating disorder.[5] *Ninety-seven* percent of women admit to having at least one "I hate my body" moment each day, although for most it's thirty-five, fifty, or even one hundred; which means that for every waking hour, the average woman will hurl between one and eight cruel insults at herself.[6]

Oh, there's more. During her lifetime, one in three women will experience sexual or physical abuse[7]; one in five women will be raped[8]; and one in four girls will be sexually abused before the age of eighteen.[9] There are 220 words for a sexually promiscuous woman but only twenty for a sexually promiscuous man.[10] Globally, there are an estimated 4.5 million people trapped in forced sexual exploitation.[11] Twenty-six percent of women between ages eighteen and twenty-four have been stalked online, and another 25 percent have been the target of online sexual harassment.[12] It is enough to douse a girl's inner fire and leave her choking on her own ashes. But you don't need two depressing paragraphs of statistics to tell you that something is very wrong here.

Add to this barrage something I call the "script": a set of harsh rules and conditions, both spoken and unspoken, which demand that you give up *who you truly are* in order to play the part of *who you are supposed to be.* You learn: *Be good. Be nice. Be pretty. Be thin. Be perfect. And whatever you do, don't be too much, too big, or too loud.* The script is a noose around the neck of your soul. While the script may differ from family to family, culture to culture, and nation to nation, it always requires you to second-guess what you innately know, and to trade what you innately want for what your family, culture, or nation wants (read: demands) of you. As your inner compass becomes no longer consultable or trustable, you do what every woman does when swimming in crazy soup for far too long: you go to war, usually against yourself. While the requirements listed in the script vary, the damage you inflict upon yourself while trying to live by the script's rules is all too familiar.

It's a man's world after all. You exist in a world that values and rewards what I call your Masculine Genius: your rational, linear, go-go-go, get-it-done, goal-oriented, competitive, will-powered abilities. It is that same world that shames and hobbles your intuitive, meaningful, collaborative, emotional, passionate, spiraling, soulful abilities—your Feminine Genius.

The script requires you to conform to a narrow and confining definition of womanhood, or to try not to appear feminine at all. If you are like the women I get to know and work with, you think that if you want to be successful, free, powerful, and strong, you should think, act, speak, decide, work, and work out more like a man. And if you want to belong, and feel valuable, lovable, and attractive, you had best nip and tuck yourself into the ideal of a woman that the dominant culture has laid out for you. So as you read this you might find yourself—as most women and many men do too—more than a touch sad, sick, and off-course.

But.

You are not crazy; it's the collective system that is out of whack. Your wildness isn't the problem; it's the cage that you put around yourself. It turns out that the serious out of whackness is "only" about five thousand years old and is neither divinely nor biologically ordained, as explains researcher and writer Riane Eisler. Eisler's research of Western archeology, social science, history, religion, and anthropology has allowed her to shed new light on the art, wall paintings, cave sanctuaries, and burial sites from roughly 2.6 million years ago through about 30 BCE, from the civilizations of the Paleolithic and Neolithic ages through those of ancient Crete and Greece. One of her works, *The Chalice and the Blade*—which explains how our current culture has evolved to hold women in such low regard—has been called by anthropologist Ashley Montagu "the most important book since Darwin's *Origin of the Species*."

Eisler found that up until about five thousand years ago, goddesses were revered alongside gods, peace was considered to be greater than war, and the life-death cycle was not seen as something to outwit or outrun, but as a powerful force to respect and revere. The fertile feminine body, the womb, and the vulva were all seen as points of worship.

Even when deities were fashioned as female, it was not that women dominated men; men and women lived as equals, neither gender being inferior nor superior. The sexual was not yet bound to the violent and dominant; the erotic was not yet separated from the sacred; and the sacred was not yet stripped from the Feminine. Fossils, bones, carvings, tools, and writings whisper to us that, once, that was simply a way of life.

how much brighter will life become when the Sacred Feminine again flourishes in us all?

THIS IS JUST THE BEGINNING

It was not until I was in my early thirties, when I was staring down retirement from my performing career in dance, that a path back to myself slowly started to appear. In need of a new way to support myself financially, I stumbled across the career path of holistic health coaching. I saw that it would allow me to be my own boss while helping other people to live, eat, and relate better. It would also allow me to heal from the physical and psychic injuries I had sustained from my lifetime of warring with myself.

What I learned to do with clients, I practiced first on myself. Along with coaching skills like high-quality questions and high-quality listening, I mastered how to decode cravings. As I examined the impulses, longings, yearnings, needs, wants, and desires I had felt my whole life—like for ice cream sundaes, skipping class, or kissing boys—I realized that each impulse was an encoded message, designed to make me aware of some physical or metaphysical nutrient I needed more of in my life, be it healthy fats, more rest, a truer connection with others, or (almost always) a truer connection with myself.

Oh, I realized, *my body doesn't lie. My wanting, longing, desirous, feeling body isn't a problem. In fact, what I want is actually key to helping me get where I want to go.*

One afternoon, I sat in a lecture on Vedic Tantric philosophy (the guiding principle behind many forms of yoga), for which I was getting certified so I could offer it to my coaching clients. Originating in India around the fifth century, the word *tantra* loosely translates as "web" or "weaving." As I learned that day, Tantrists—an unruly band of mystical upstarts—believe that since all life is interconnected (like a web), humans are not separate from God (or whatever term you choose for the divine power that animates all of life), but are in fact interwoven with God.

Many world religions see humans as inherently and irreparably flawed, salvageable only if we live precisely by one ordained script or another, getting high enough marks in this lifetime to earn our reunion with All That Is in some kind of afterlife. Tantrism, however, like the Buddhism and Hinduism it influenced, sees humans as suffering only from a simple, easily reparable misunderstanding. We aren't separate from the Holy One; we have simply *forgotten* that the Holy One and we are one. We aren't hopelessly messed up; we have simply *forgotten* that the Divine is having a messy human experience through us. We needn't follow a stringent set of conditions in order to be worthy of love; we have simply *forgotten* that the Universe adores us unconditionally. Tantra kindly reminds us that whatever it is we have simply forgotten, we can remember.

Oh, I realized. *So, I am a strand in the web of All That Is. That means that no matter how many pounds I gain, classes I flunk, or relationships I mess up, I will still get an A+ from the Universe.*

It slowly dawned on me that if being human is not a fallen condition, neither is being a woman. No longer my prosecutor and executioner, my hunger became holy. Instead of hurling my requisite one hundred "I hate my body" bombs at myself each day, I realized that—as a woman and a human—I could sing a new refrain to myself. I repeated a line from Mary Oliver's poem "Wild Geese": "You only have to let the soft animal of your body love what it loves." I began to see that no script could ever teach me how to be the woman I was aching to become, nor could it ever teach me how to truly feel, speak, work, love, or know myself as holy. No script could—but my body, my soul, and I could.

As I built my coaching practice—learning and growing and falling and failing—something surprising happened. My new career slowly became a calling. Really. Feminine Genius herself (although at the time I didn't call her that or really know what she was) kept calling me and whispering, *Steady on. Women are the key.* The wild grace of Feminine Genius blossomed in my body like spring-drunk forsythia and refused to ever let me go. Feminine Genius directed my wary gaze onto a path that curved off into a future that didn't at all resemble my scripted, contorted past. Then without any instruction, Feminine Genius cackled a bit, smacked me on the ass, and sent me walking.

So, for the past fourteen years, I have supported women from all over the globe, from more than fifty countries and six continents. I have worked with hundreds in individual coaching sessions and live retreats, and with thousands through digital courses and my online community. My job description, as I see it, is to help women flourish in this world, a world in which the opposite of flourishing is too often the norm. As you and I go along through these pages, I will share about my clients, readers, friends, participants, colleagues, and mentors so that you can see how this Feminine Genius stuff has been of use not just to me but also to real-life, flesh-and-blood women worldwide.

One of the most enduringly inspiring things in my life is to watch a woman slip the Gordian knot of self-loathing, people pleasing, and overachieving and become simply and fully herself. The light that comes on in her, comes on in the world; it confirms that I am doing my part to leave this wacky world that much better than I found it, one Feminine Genius at a time.

> One is not born a genius, one becomes a genius; and the feminine situation has up to the present rendered this becoming practically impossible.
> **SIMONE DE BEAUVOIR**, *The Second Sex*

2

The Provocative Path
Where I'm Leading You

For the things we have to learn before we can do them,
we learn by doing them.
ARISTOTLE, *Nichomachean Ethics*

It turns out there is a path to help you become the woman you are aching to become.

This path is well worn and always brings you home, but please do not mistake it for a script, a map, or a blueprint.

This path is provocative, just as the title of this book suggests. This path is unruly, messy, and a wee bit naughty, and audaciously asks you to trust the very parts of yourself that you previously warred against. This path demands that as you stride into your own bright life, instead of using a script, map, or blueprint, you use your sensuous, desirous, wildly feeling female body as a steadfast and trustworthy compass. (Which may at first sound like blasphemy, but I assure you can actually be gospel. "Good," "orderly," and "perfect" are so last century, anyway.)

So be forewarned: this path is highly nonconformist, requires boat-loads of moxie, and will be relayed by a provocateur in hiking boots without a money-back guarantee. Nice to meet you, I'm LiYana, and I'll be your gospel-singing, hiking-booted Sherpa on this path for the next 250 or so pages.

I was not born with the reverence and respect I now have for femininity. I had to learn it, lose it, re-learn it, and recover it. I had to fall, fail, flail, and rise again. More times than I was comfortable with, honestly. I am not about to reveal some conspiracy theory. There are not (for the most part) armies of men out there, waiting to do you in. Nor is the trick to simply kick your masculine strengths to the curb and *be more feminine*. I want to re-introduce you to your often maligned and ignored feminine strengths so that you can integrate them with your already awesome masculine strengths. For these reasons, and more, I like to think that I make quite a trusty—albeit unorthodox—tour guide on the path of Feminine Genius.

This path is one to becoming fully yourself: feeling at home in your skin and gloriously sexy. Connecting to a deeper sense of why you are here and what you are called to contribute. Wise, bold choice making. A rich sensual life. Profound intimacy. Creative fire. Deep strength. Epic love.

Passion. Grace. Humility and wild abandon.

Confidence—the untamable kind.

This path requires you, as it has required me, to use a radical and new lens with which to see yourself. To see that your face is the face of the Goddess. That your ups and downs are a not a sickness and that your sexuality is not dangerous. That there is a kernel of wisdom inside every one of your demons. That your impulses, intuitions, and longings are how the Holy One has a word with you.

As you get the hang of using this lens, you will see that your body is not evidence of your fall from grace; it is actually your very portal to the Divine. That your desires aren't saboteurs; they can actually act like fertilizer, growing your wisdom. That you can express your desires in a way that has others excited to help you meet them. That you can surf and sail your emotions, rather than be sunk by them. That inner peace doesn't just come through calming your mind, but also through shakin' what your mama gave you. That you can—and must—loosen any energy blocks you may have developed from years of holding back your truth, and seal up any energy leaks you might have developed from years of fearing other women as the enemy.

This path asks of you, as it asks of me, to take on an often counterintuitive set of life practices so that you can thrive magnificently in
a world built for the Masculine Genius in all of us. And in doing so,
re-create the world as one that works for men and women alike, which
is a mission particularly suited to Feminine Genius. Our collective,
crazy, war-torn past need not become your future. It won't, unless you
authorize it.

*This, Beloved, is a most auspicious
Time To be a woman*

So, wherever you are in the world and wherever you are on your personal journey, welcome. You are welcome here. I wrote this for *you*.

Whether you are a soaring entrepreneur or an aspiring student, an
established exec or mover and shaker, a hopeful mother or a deter-
mined wife, an intellectual or an artist, a ladder-climber or spiritual
seeker (or a bit of each), allow me to embolden you to turn down
the volume on everyone else's advice, shred the script you have been
handed, and learn to source your guidance and wisdom from within.
Let me offer you this book to use as your walking staff as you stride
down the path into a brilliant (although imperfect) life that is your
destiny and legacy.

> A book must be the axe for the frozen sea inside us.
> **FRANZ KAFKA**

A deep bow to you for picking up the axe. You are extraordinary and
brave and radical and my heroine for being here. For the sliver of
geography in every woman that is frozen, let me offer some mouth-to-
mouth resuscitation for your light and heat—that magnificence that
gushes free when you ruthlessly swing the axe and gently turn yourself

back on. In a world that will tell you ten thousand times a day you are wrong, I will unflinchingly remind you, in a thousand different ways, of your rightness.

As I see it, women are like candle flames: dazzling sources of light and fire. But most of us are dimmed way down. Barely a flicker. When I try to count the collective woman-hours we spend self-bashing and attempting to become superwomen—or men—I realize I can't count that high.

What might be possible if those woman-hating woman-hours were diverted and instead channeled into a healthy body, a healthy mind, a reinvigorated sex life, a true sense of self-love, an act of creativity, a consciously created family, a new business, a community service? As I see it, the root cause of the world's suffering is that women are dimmed down, stressed-out, and burned-out. The woman who will help to light, lead, and heal our world does the radical act of turning her own inner flame back on.

This path is designed to give you just what you need so you can: Turn. Yourself. Back. On.

Do you know what a woman feels like, awake and fully thawed?

As seeker—looking God in the eye in the bathroom mirror. Loving this life that has met you at your razor's edge and tossed you over that edge, as only a holy trickster can.

As mother—playful and present. Modeling for the next generation what you now know to be true about a woman's body, feelings, longings, and divinity.

As lover—sensually alive and communing. A living, breathing temple to ecstasy, to discovering facets of yourself you never knew existed, wielding your unvarnished, untarnished, divine, healing power.

As leader—deeply in love with those you serve. Whether one-on-one or to multitudes, contributing meaningfully to the world, without burning out.

As friend—vulnerable, brave, and bold. Speaking up, getting lit off another's brilliance, and then passing along the favor the next chance you get.

Can you picture a world filled with this kind of woman?

I can. (Hint: she looks like you.)

So let me take you now, before the gangrene of this crazy world does.

It is the world that's nutso, woman, not you. You are right as rain. The power that attracts metal filings to a magnet is the same power that surges through your belly. The wisdom that lets the cherry trees know when to burst into bloom is the same wisdom that runs through your veins. The light that a candle spreads over a dusky room is the same light that shines from your eyes. The brilliance that funded Einstein is waiting for you, Feminine Genius.

The world may have simply forgotten how wise, clear, powerful, and magical you are. But I have not.

And you, too, can remember.

your body never lies
your hunger is holy
your truth is a direct line to the Divine
what you deeply desire
will lead you into the life you were
born to live
and will require you
to become the woman you are
aching to become

WHERE AM I TAKING YOU?

As you lace up your walking boots and get ready to take your first steps onto this provocative path, let me give you your general itinerary. In the next two chapters of part one, Going to the Source, I will show you where the trouble starts for too many girls and young women, a place in time when your power may have lessened but where your life story can start to be powerfully rewritten. And then it is time to say hello to Feminine Genius herself. It's darn near impossible to capture this force of nature in a single sound bite, so you'll have to join me in that chapter where we will go right to the Source.

The rest of this book—part discourse, part workbook, part story, part hymnal—is divided into three more parts, Navigating Your Dark, Embodying Your Genius, and Cultivating Your Light.

Navigating Your Dark

I deliberately head straight into the dark stuff because I stand for the underdog and underbelly in us all. I find that there is nothing like your dark—a storm of "negative" emotions, a long streak of "bad luck," or the crumbling of your world—to stop you in your tracks or make you turn on yourself. If you can make it through your dark, you can make it anywhere.

You probably don't yet know that your *shadow* is simply parts of yourself you haven't met yet. Waiting in your dark is a shaft of light pointing you toward your next move. The dark is not punishment for being weak; it holds the keys to your strength. The dark is not a step off your path; it is an integral part of your journey. The dark forges the lead of your doubts into the gold of your courage. Once you learn how to navigate the underworld of the unknown, it becomes impossible to feel truly forsaken, ever again.

Embodying Your Genius

Allow me to re-introduce you to some forgotten truths: Your mind is not the smartest thing about you; your body is wildly intelligent.

Your body is not an impediment to divinity; your body *is* divine. Your passion, intuition, and inspiration for what you came here to do, this call and response with whatever you call God, is a language you can learn. The mouthpiece for this mother tongue is right in your body, albeit in an unlikely location.

The very things you have assumed will ruin you—your impulses, urges, desires, and erotic energy—are actually designed to reconnect you with your life-force and holy fire. When understood and integrated into your psyche, these truths help you embody your wisdom and guide you home.

Cultivating Your Light

As I see it, women are made to burn bright. In this final section, I lay out mindsets and practices to help you keep your flame lit in a world that tends to dim you. So that you can re-learn why divine guidance is best heard when you are turned on. So that you can re-forge the connection of your pleasure to your confidence. So that you can use your ups as well as your downs to feel more powerfully present and alive. So that you can boldly express your desires, and fully receive them when they come.

So that, as you bring your Feminine Genius into your friendships, relationships, and everyday life, you can lay a path of light through the darkness in our world.

HOW TO SUCK THE MARROW OUT OF THESE PAGES

You picked up this book. You want significant change. Here's how you can fully absorb the wisdom here and make it yours.

Do the Practices

Your body's wisdom is not found through conceptual thought or through contemplating philosophies. Your inner knowing is not sourced through thinking deeply on theoretical hypotheses. Your confidence, clarity, and creativity are not static concepts. Each arises as an unmistakable felt sense from your actual physical body.

So, please, toss your blood-and-bone self into the laboratory of trial and error, trial and error, trial and error. Try things on and see how they fit before you decide they are—or are not—for you. And as you follow the "letter of the law" in trying out the practices as I have laid them out, please also drink in the "spirit of the law," and transmute my intentions into your own lawless authority.

When You Have an *Aha!* Moment, Record It

A journal is a great way to record your insights. My favorite is sticky notes. The inside of your arm (or thigh) will do in a pinch, as will the virgin margins of this book. But, here's why: each *aha!* is a light bulb of insight that your inner genius switched on just for you. Each *aha!* is a tiki torch shedding some light on your trail as you walk.

So take note. Nail those suckers to the wall. They are slippery little buggers, so it's good to pin them down with pen and ink. Greedily gather these breadcrumbs on the path to your becoming fully yourself.

Should You Skip Around or Read from Beginning to End?

Great question. I wrote this book so that you could, starting with your big toe, slowly and incrementally submerge your whole wise body in these hot waters without suddenly scalding yourself. That's the compelling case for starting on page one and proceeding in an orderly fashion to the end.

However, I love rebels. If you choose the haphazard route, I suggest you treat each non sequitur nugget you come across as medicine. Let it blaze in your belly, light you up like a firecracker, and burn away all that no longer serves you.

And I suggest you don't make your way through this book entirely alone. For practices and resources that were too rebellious to be included here, and for my guidelines for forming a book club so you can walk this provocative path with a few fellow Feminine Geniuses, come find me at liyanasilver.com/bookresources.

Terms of Engagement

This is a book about the biggies: your body, soul, and inner knowing; about women, intelligence, desire, sex, God, and power. Somewhere in here, if not on every page, I am bound to smack one of your sacred cows right between the eyes. I speak frankly about women's experiences, many of which are, frankly, heartbreaking. But since I don't think polite silence or tidy language serves anyone, my cow-smacking frankness is a good thing, I promise. If a term I use doesn't work for you, swap it out for one of your own that does. Just stay with me.

And listen, although I love the rigors of research as much as the next goddess, I ultimately care less about what some study "proves" than what the hallowed halls of your mind, heart, and body know is true. Honestly, sometimes I wish that my task of reuniting a woman with her truth was easier, neater, and less controversial, but what's a gal to do? This is no time for the faint of heart. Everything is at stake. Someone has to say it so that you can live life on your own terms.

Wake Up, Every Day

Instead of shutting yourself up in an ashram, university, or convent, this path demands that you throw open the gates and welcome in your stinky, quirky, workaday life. This path says that even your lust, wrath, and greed can help you to awaken. This path asks that you intermingle the sacred and mundane so that the ordinary becomes the extraordinary. As author Mirabai Starr says, "Our greatest sages do not bail out of this world; they embrace it. Enlightened beings become more human, not less. They too crave chocolate, they wake up in bad moods, they flirt at parties. They are *us*."[1]

Wake up, sage.

Will This Work for You?

This material has been culled from over fourteen years of my work with women, and has proven useful for me, for readers, for clients, for participants, and for friends. However, I would never presume to know what is best for every woman. It is my sincere prayer, as you tuck into these pages, that you feel my reverence for your unique story and that you unearth for yourself a gem—or ten.

I have never come across a woman who truly wanted to find her way back to herself, who didn't. And, sister, if that is what you want, I want that for you. So much, in fact, that I wrote you a freakin' book. So, give it a whirl. And for the love of all that is holy, track me down and share with me how you made it work for yourself.

Whatever You Do, Use It

Use this book as a set of coordinates to find your own way home. Chew it and swallow it whole. Get blood on your chin. Dog-ear the pages, rip sections out and post them on your bathroom wall, highlight passages that sing in your ears. Please don't contemplate it passively like an innocent bystander. Don't use it as an expensive paperweight or let it gather dust on your nightstand. Use it up. This book will alter forever the course of your woman's life, if you let it.

Let it.

fiercely embodying the Sacred Feminine
is a process of coming home
as well as becoming home
welcome home, woman
welcome home.

3

My Story, Our Story
Where, Oh Where, Did Our Power Go?

Broken is the beginning.
GLENNON DOYLE MELTON

t usually happens first in girlhood: a break, a crack, a violation, a rupture, a slow, molten erosion—or many of them. Whether intentional or accidental, whether at the hands of caretakers or through the influence of media or culture—or the girl or boy next door—you, as a girl child, had formative early experiences that stole a bit of your fire, and dented, wounded, and bent you out of shape.

Based on those experiences, you developed painful, restrictive beliefs about yourself, about other people, and about life itself. These restrictive beliefs do a great job of, well, restricting you. They hide your light under a bushel. However, these restrictive beliefs are simply "act 1," the first vignette of your life's story.

As painful as they are, these beliefs need not determine what kind of present moment you live in or destiny you walk into. As impossible as it may at first seem, you can alchemize the leaden beliefs of your past into your own hand-forged golden future. The wild and wise girl child that you may have thought was lost can rise again. Helping you rewrite act 1, with yourself as the heroine of a captivating play, is one thing that the Sacred Feminine is—honestly—genius at. The rest of this chapter—and this book—is about rewriting those beliefs so you can let your light shine.

Rewriting your beliefs changes your day-to-day experience of yourself, of your life, and of others. In turn, it changes your behaviors, and trickles down and changes your biochemistry, so that the thoughts you think, the actions you take, and the feelings you feel, change forever and for good. So that what you know to be true about yourself, life, and others changes forever and for good. You bow to your broken beginning and turn to stride into the rest your life.

But, oh, act 1 can be so hard and heavy.

WHAT GOES ON — AND WHAT GOES WRONG — IN ACT 1

Rose came to one of my retreats, fresh off an airplane from her home in Australia where she runs a thriving business and raises her son and daughter. Rose's mother was Maori, the indigenous tribe of New Zealand, and was only seventeen years old when she left Rose's biological father to get Rose away from what had become a physically and emotionally abusive relationship. At twenty-one, in need of food, clothes, and shelter, Rose's mother married again.

Rose was a twelve-year-old on the cusp of womanhood the first time her stepfather touched her, and his molestation continued until she was sixteen. Rose was on constant high alert for all of those years, and many times begged her mother to leave him and take her and her two half sisters away. But even though her mother hated living that life, she didn't take them away. In fact, her mother eventually made Rose leave home to keep the peace.

Rose began to believe that it was no longer safe for her to know what she knew, that being a girl was dangerous, and that being a woman meant being in bondage. She tucked away part of her power into a secret fold of her psyche. As Rose separated herself from her girlhood, she also separated herself from what she felt were weak and untrustworthy "feminine" aspects she saw in her mother and in herself. Naturally fierce, intuitive, and deeply connected with the natural world, Rose's girlhood spirit was clipped and pruned, then fenced off.

Rose became a successful entrepreneur, supporting other women in their creativity and self-expression, but she also worked all the time, was often exhausted, found it hard to rest, felt competitive with her colleagues, and secretly doubted that she was making a difference for anyone. Rose did a version of what most women do in order to survive in a "man's world"—she put her head down, put part of herself aside, and made something of herself—but not without sacrificing her full radiance.

Baby, It's a Man's World

Rose's beginning is a dramatic version of how girlhood goes for too many: your shameless joy for being alive gets rudely interrupted, and your unassailable internal knowing ebbs as you cross into womanhood.

In a thousand ways, from birth to death and every day in between, everything that could be wrong with you—as a girl and as a woman—gets listed, repeated, regurgitated, and burned into your bones. Even if your act 1 was less traumatic or dramatic than Rose's, you were probably still handed a how-to-be-happy script with nifty little check boxes for the perfect body, partner, job, faith, house, and shoes. But as you know all too well, following a script is trip-wired. It requires you to mistrust the impulses of your body, to misunderstand your intuitive guidance, and malign your deepest desires. It requires you to war with yourself and other women.

It is stressful to be on a crusade against your body, your psyche, and your fellow humans. Chronic stress—be it physical, psychological, or spiritual—causes chronic inflammation in your body, and is the root cause of not only depression but also the biggest physical health challenges facing women: heart disease, Alzheimer's, and cancer. Many scientific studies are done on male subjects (human or animal) so that the results aren't "skewed" by menstruation, so you often receive medical perspectives that are best suited for a 160-pound male.

In a world designed more with men, maleness, and masculinity in mind, you develop a feeling that something is fundamentally wrong and flawed within you, within your femaleness. You grow to assume that someone else—be that person a doctor, rabbi, priest, parent, expert, or Oprah herself—knows better than you do. You get the message that you will become more spiritual (or enlightened) only by ignoring, purifying, or transcending your body. You learn that it is virtuous to cultivate a calm (and positive) mind and triumph over your messy emotions. You learn to smile, look pretty, and pretend you don't feel dark, distressed, or depleted.

In order to "make it" in a world more suited to masculine models of success, sexuality, spirituality, and professionalism, you overuse your masculine strengths, becoming gravely out of alignment with your feminine cycles. You "make it" by medicating your moods, caffeinating your productivity, stifling your voice, dumbing down your sensuality, and trying to beat out the competition. When you falter or flag, perpetually one accessory shy of perfection, you pull yourself up by your bootstraps and re-enter the battle with renewed determination.

In trying to be superwoman, supermom, or superworker, you fry your adrenals, choke your thyroid gland, become utterly depleted, get into painful competition with other women, question your purpose (and worth) on the planet, and dry up below the waist.

Most leaders, decision makers, and folks in power, even the few that are women, don't look particularly sensually alive; at the same time, most of us understand that a woman's sexuality is a hot commodity that can sell, buy, or get nearly anything. So you do your damnedest to appear sexy, but not too sexy, because you also know that your sexuality can be used against you to cheapen, defile, and dirty you.

You learn to use your sexuality as a weapon or a currency, or you ignore it completely and pretend to be chaste and professional. Since one in three women will be sexually abused or violated in her lifetime, any confusion you have about your sexuality and power is (unfortunately) quite normal.

One in three. Pause for a second.

Look around. Can you see (or imagine) three women? One of those women has had or will have her sexual innocence prematurely snatched from her. She might do the near impossible and pry back from the jaws of death an appreciation for her body, a feeling of general physical safety, and a robust trust for sensual energy, but it is less common than we would wish it to be. If she can once again feel at home in her skin, she will be the exception, not the rule.

Look around. Can you see (or imagine) two women? Count yourself in as the third, because that third woman, that one in three from the faceless statistic I just quoted, might just wear your face.

There are as many different beliefs as there are people, all with an astounding level of nuance and individuality. But over my fourteen years of helping to make sense of seemingly senseless act 1s and helping to rewrite restrictive beliefs through a process I call "belief re-patterning" in client sessions, leading groups, and interacting with readers, there are four main groups of restrictive beliefs that rise to the top of the fray. The first group of hard and heavy beliefs comes straight out of my own act 1.

ACT 1, REVISITED

My parents rarely raised their voices or fought. But on one particular snowy night, I wondered, a slow creep of doubt across my belly, if something was wrong. My four-year-old ears noted that my dad's voice was brittle, alarming, and full of sharp edges as he watched my mom put our dinner of spaghetti and tomato sauce on the round wooden kitchen table.

Suddenly, my dad grabbed the edge of the table and gave it a powerful heave. I froze while the whole kitchen exploded into brimstone and chaos. Broken shards of plates stabbed the guts of the noodles and lodged in the blood of the sauce. My mom said nothing. She put on her snow boots, slammed out the front door, and disappeared into the black night, all but brushing shrapnel off her shoulders as she went.

A tiny crack appeared in my frozen brain, and a painful belief seared like lightening: *Anger breaks things. Conflict makes people leave. Things can break without warning. If I don't fix it, I will be left. Forever. Go. Fix it. Now.*

That was the moment I started to become a conflict-fixing, people-pleasing perfectionist. Perfectionism, a form of people pleasing, is a compulsion to paper over a deep mistrust in yourself and in life, like slapping a Band-Aid over the warning light of a car dashboard. That was the moment I began to believe that harmony is more valuable than expressing a need or yelping honestly in pain. That saying the "right" thing is more important than saying what I feel is true. That others can't handle what they feel; I must do it for them. That emotional upset equals abandonment and must be "fixed" immediately before it can irreparably snap human connection like a twig.

That winter night, so long ago, I put on my own tiny snow boots and all but leaped through the snow drifts after my mom, my little legs struggling to make it from one mommy-boot-shaped trench to another. I found her a half mile up our driveway and vaulted into her arms, my landing pad the startling cold of her down jacket. At once hysterical and focused, I touched her face and applied my four-year-old diplomacy: "Mommy, can we go back now? Mommy, please, let's go home."

And we did. The windows were wide-eyed and glowing from the inside. And inside, slowly, silently, sheepishly, my dad picked splinters out of the viscera of our cold spaghetti dinner.

Formative beliefs take hold in a moment where your sense of love, belonging, or survival seem threatened. This holds true even if—as in my case—the upsetting incident was fairly uncommon. I didn't grow up in a household riddled with conflict. But still, on that long-ago winter night, my lifelong aversion to conflict and my long-suffering case of perfectionism was formed. From that night onward, like too many women do, I trained myself to detect the moment that my anger (or any other emotion that could spark dispute) sprang into being, and I would swallow it whole. Like too many women do, I stole away with my truth and sacrificed it to the gods of perfection.

And, while I could tell "perfect" was going to be a lot of work, I knew I was just the young woman for the job. I graduated high school as valedictorian, spent weeknights and weekends rehearsing for dance and theatre productions, and got into every prestigious college I applied to—and I applied to ten. If there were odds to be found, I wanted to beat them, no matter what I had to do to myself in the process. I became addicted to overworking and under-earning and to overwhelm and under-eating. I refused to recognize much more than a tiny bit of my own success, value, or beauty. After all, I was not yet perfect.

Yes, I am unique, and my act 1 experiences are unique, but nearly every woman I come across has a version of the belief I formed on that snowy evening of spaghetti death: "Me? I don't need help. I've got it, don't worry! I'm a giver; I was put on this Earth to give and give and give. I have to do it all by myself. No one is going to do it as good or fast as me, anyway. But once I have over-done, over-given, and over-achieved for long enough, perhaps you'll consider loving me in return. How does that sound as a deal?"

And thus, as a result of an act 1 sort of like mine, **Restrictive Beliefs Group #1** is formed and goes something like this: *Needs make you weak. Get rid of all needs. Ask for nothing; take nothing. Get busy giving and doing—but make sure you do it all by yourself. I can't need much because I don't deserve much. I am a mistake. I am not wanted. I don't deserve to be here. I have to earn my existence.*

Act 1 for Callie, one of my mentees, began when she turned five, and her friend and neighbor, eight years older than her, started touching her. When Callie and I began working together in a group program on women's embodiment, she was thirty-five years old, a statuesque, whip-smart, self-employed project manager. I loved how we often spoke of fairies, homemade blackberry jam, and computer code all in the same few minutes. Callie was in a fourteen-year relationship that everyone assumed would turn into marriage and last a lifetime, but Callie was increasingly, alarmingly, unsure. She wanted to do everything she could—personal growth, looking at her own demons, working on her communication and sex life with her partner—so she could answer for herself one of the hardest questions, "Should I stay or should I go? And how will I know?"

But back on her family's farm (literally, Callie's girlhood was spent on a hobby farm in Northern California), five-year-old Callie had gone along with what her friend and neighbor suggested they do and try. After all, he was older and she trusted him. Callie was at first curious about the new energy and sensations she experienced with him, but over the coming months, it all started to feel "off." So, one day she barged in on her mother making lunch, laid out what was happening with the neighbor kid, and asked what she should do about it.

This clear and empowered girl child's question did not go over well. Not at all. Callie could tell by her mother's stiffening body that something had just gone very, very wrong. Confused, Callie struggled to understand what she had done to make her mother so cold. Her mother told Callie to stop making things up, that the neighbor boy would never do anything like that, and that "good girls don't get into situations like that."

Callie's inner mouth clamped shut. Her ability to speak up disappeared. There in the pantry of her childhood home, holding on to her mother's apron strings, she began to believe, *Sexual energy is dangerous. My body is dirty and wrong. I don't have a voice. I can't trust anyone to really keep me safe and care for me.*

You can follow Callie's belief train, right? If good girls don't get into situations like that, it stands to reason that she must not be a good girl. The opposite of a good girl is a dirty and wrong girl. Situations "like that," with sexual energy present, must be avoided upon penalty of removal of Mother's love. And as for speaking up and saying it like it is? As Callie tried to ask for help to get out of an increasingly unwanted situation, she was told she was a liar. It was no longer safe for her to feel what she felt. Her trust in others to help keep her safe broke.

As she crossed into womanhood, Callie became chronically anxious about sex. Throughout her years of partnership, she often felt numb to her partner's touch and resented him for trying to connect intimately with her. She tried to express to him what she wanted and what he could do or say that would have her feel more open to him, but they both got frustrated when he didn't understand how. Callie trusted almost no one to have her best interests at heart. She was plagued by ambivalence, wondering if she should keep working on herself and her "issues" or whether she was with the wrong guy and should do them both a favor, call a spade a spade, and move on.

An act 1 sort of like Callie's helps to form **Restrictive Beliefs Group #2**: *I can't trust my body. I can't trust other people. My body will betray me.*

I am weak; I am broken; I am damaged goods. I can't trust sexual energy. Desire and pleasure will get me into trouble.

Riya, whom I got to know through our individual coaching sessions and group retreats, infuses warmth and sparkle into any room she enters. A lawyer, wife to a Fortune 500 executive, and mother of a teenage son, Riya also moonlights as a priestess. For real. Riya tracks down wise spiritual mentors in obscure towns and travels tenaciously to study with them and absorb their wisdom.

In one of our sessions, we traced back to one of Riya's original ruptures in her act 1. Riya was four, standing up in the backseat of the family car, gripping the faux leather headrest to steady herself, talking and singing excitedly at the top of her mini lungs. Face tight with annoyance, her aunt turned around and said, "Riya, you're talking too much. Will someone give her some food to quiet her down?"

Riya's song stopped. Tiny wheels began to turn in Riya's heart. As it sank in that her "too loud" voice and "too big" presence was a problem—a big problem, a too big problem—a belief formed: *Who I am, as I am, is too much. So I will be who they want me to be, so they will love me.*

Riya began to try to tone down her boldness and loudness. The voices of her mother, father, aunts, uncles, and grandparents in her Indian-American family became louder than her own inner voice. For this naturally precocious, vivacious little girl who naturally knew her own mind, it became harder and harder to hear what she wanted for herself, until eventually she couldn't go there at all. Her inner voice simmered down, and then went mute.

Although she was of average weight, Riya became obsessed with being thinner and more beautiful. Throughout college and the early days of her marriage, she would sneak cigarettes and binge on junky foods in order to calm her nerves and "quiet herself down." She would then take all the evidence down to the trash bins behind the house before her husband got home. A chasm formed between them. After her Monday through Friday routine of dieting, fighting with her husband, sneaking food, and working a job she barely tolerated, on weekend nights she would go out dancing and drinking with friends to "let off steam."

This went on for about ten years until one Friday night she rearended a car. Looking at the driving-under-the-influence ticket in her shaking hands, Riya realized that she could have just killed someone. She realized that the part of her that she was stuffing down in order to make her family happy had burst out of its seams and could have taken two lives with it. She felt the cold, hard floor of her personal rock bottom smack her in the face.

Restrictive Beliefs Group #3 comes from an act 1 sort of like Riya's: *I'm not enough. I'm too much. I feel too much. I am too loud, too big, too bold. I am not lovable as I am. I can't do what I want and still be accepted. I always make the wrong choice. I must be perfect. I can't speak up, or I will lose love. What I have to say doesn't matter. I don't have a voice.*

Remember Rose, the beautiful Maori warrioress from the beginning of this chapter? Rose's act 1 beliefs—about womanhood as indentured servitude, and about colleagues as competition—bring it all full circle and complete the set, with **Restrictive Beliefs Group #4:** *It is not safe to see what I see. It is not safe to know what I know. I don't know enough. Others know better than me. The only way to be free is to not be me.*

Ours are four unique childhood stories, yet I see our stories and our resultant beliefs repeated, in infinite variation, in the women I get to work with, as well as in my friends and colleagues. (You may have found some of your own beliefs in there, I suspect.)

These ever popular, restrictive beliefs effectively separate you from your own truth, voice, and sense of personal power. You might then tend to lose yourself in relationships, mothering, achievement, work, or "keeping up with the Joneses," and might often lead a secret life, where you can express aspects of your true self on the sly, often with unhealthy and dangerous side effects.

Rewriting Your Beliefs with Feminine Genius

That's the bad news. Ready for the good news?

Instead of going on to live numb lives, unhappy or cut off from our power, each of us—myself, Rose, Callie, and Riya—came to a reckoning point. We each took a deep breath and took the path less traveled, a path that routed us through our shadow—that place in our psyche that holds our unwanted, unknown, and outdated beliefs. Wild and winding, the path eventually brought us back to our body, our voice, our girlhood, our womanhood, and our native intrepidity, innocence, and genius. The cracks are, to borrow from the songwriter Leonard Cohen, how the light gets in.

The reckoning point is when you see that there is a problem in your life, yet you refuse to cast yourself or anyone else as the villain. You want to change but, to paraphrase Einstein, you know that trying to solve any problem with the same reasoning that created the problem is insanity. At the reckoning point, you notice the particular kind of box you are in, and you lift the lid of that box and climb out so that you can begin to think "outside the box."

As I see it, in order to rewrite your restrictive beliefs (and the script you learned to follow as a result) and forge a new future for yourself, you must resist focusing forever on what your parents or caregivers did or didn't do. As I see it, on a metaphysical level, we have all tasked our families and life journeys to repeatedly gift us with yet another chance to learn and to grow. (Or, to put it less politely as my acronym-loving, spaghetti-tossing dad would: AFGO—Another Fucking Growth Opportunity.)

As intense, random, and rude as your growth opportunities can be, I know it can be hard to see them as intentional—and even loving—parts of the grand design of your life. I know that your growth opportunities generally feel nearly impossible to make it through. And yet, making it through to a truer and freer version of yourself allows you to raise your face to the sky in relief and ecstasy, learned, wise, and re-united with your power. Even so, you can't rest there for long. Soon, the cycle of learning and growing begins again. (Don't blame me; take it up with Feminine Genius herself, the grand designer of your life.)

Learning to see that while your beginning might be fractured, you are never broken is pure Feminine Genius in action. Learning to see your own act 1 as a valid and valuable first step on your divine path is key to rewriting your future. You can see each subsequent growth opportunity as another lap on the cycle of learning and growing. Then, like we four women in this chapter did, you can change where you are headed, forever and for good.

Whereas Rose used to believe that being a woman was a prison sentence, she now knows that her Feminine Genius is the source of her inspirations for her life and business. Where she used to believe that creating anything would require soul-sucking toil, she now knows that she can enjoy herself and have fun as she strives. Whereas she used to feel profound self-doubt, she now knows, as you will come to know, that following someone else's map only gets her further off her path.

Whereas I used to believe that I would only be loved and accepted when I was perfect, I now know that the true measure of success is threefold: how vibrantly and sensually alive I am, how clearly I can hear my inner voice, and how much courage I have to follow my inner voice. I now know that there is wisdom in every rage, rupture, and breakdown. Thus, I no longer rob my—or anyone else's—dignity by trying to sanitize and anesthetize every conflict. I now know, as you will come to know, that welcoming these shadowy demons into the most tender part of my heart will, without fail, leave me stronger, sovereign, and more loving.

Whereas Riya used to believe that her bold, authentic self was too much, she now knows that she is more than enough. She now knows that she will only feel lovable, through and through, when she is herself, through and through. She now knows that she has everything she needs within her. She now knows, as you will come to know, that she is whole and she is home.

Whereas Callie used to believe her sexuality was toxic, she now knows that her body is sacred, and that her erotic energy is the ultimate creative force. She now knows how to radiate her beauty to inspire reverence and can choose to become invisible to unwanted, predatory energy. She now knows that her real choice (whether to stay or to go) will be made before, beyond, and in spite of reasons—and never because of reasons, no matter how compelling the reasons may be. She now knows, as you will come to know, that her body never lies and her inner knowing always guides her right into her brilliant life.

Where did your power go? Your power went running for its life after your childhood cracked, after your act 1 was interrupted. Your power went underground into your shadows as you galloped off to find a script to follow. Your power went dark as you waged a war on yourself, became deaf to your voice, and numb to your desires. Your power shape-shifted into a block of lead, waiting for you to place it in your crucible and transmute it into gold. Your power stole away into the dark night, waiting for you to welcome yourself home.

But really, prodigal daughter, your power didn't *go* anywhere. It has been here all along. Your power is waiting for you, in the most unlikely of places in your life and in the most unlikely of places in your body.

And without a doubt, sister, it is yours if you want it.

> You can start with nothing.
> And out of nothing, and out of no way,
> a way will be made.
> **REVEREND MICHAEL BERNARD BECKWITH**

4

Hello, Feminine Genius
Time to Meet Your Maker

Cease trying to work everything out with your mind.
It will get you nowhere. Live by intuition and
inspiration and let your whole life be Revelation.
EILEEN CADDY

It's about time for me to properly introduce you to Feminine Genius, wouldn't you agree? To truly convey what Feminine Genius is, I will need to mix a bit of poetry with anthropomorphism, a bit of fact with metaphor, and a bit of science with theology—but who said there must be a distinction anyway?

As I am fond of saying, a woman is like a light bulb: bright, strong, and luminous when she is turned on. So if a woman is the light bulb, then Feminine Genius is the energy that surges through the power lines, electric sockets, wires, and filaments, allowing that light bulb—or woman—to illuminate the room.

Feminine Genius is the light, and is also the woman who is lit. Feminine Genius is the power, and is also the woman who is empowered. Feminine Genius made you, and in turn, it also lets you make life. Feminine Genius is the energy of the Divine, and it is also the woman embodying the Divine.

When you dim yourself down, or the world does it for you, you likely feel cut off from your power source because you are—cut off from your Source.

Feminine Genius is Source energy—the source of light and the source of life—and is distinctly feminine and distinctly genius. Let me say more about why.

WHY "FEMININE"?

Borrowing from Vedic Tantric philosophy, I say that Source energy (or life-force, God consciousness, the Universe, or whatever term you choose for the divine power that animates all of life)—in order to know itself, experience itself, and play with itself—divided itself into two flavors of energy: one masculine and one feminine. These two flavors meet, merge, and play inside you, between you and another, and in the world at large. While every human body has Divine Masculine and Divine Feminine energies animating them, the energy of the Divine Feminine and the body of a woman have been overlooked, underplayed, and undervalued for too long.

The feminine flavor of the Divine allows us to feel, not just think; to intuit, not just reason; to be inspired, not just be productive; to want it, not just will it; to enjoy the journey, not just get to the goal; to create life, not just contain it; and to make life meaningful, not just manageable.

Metaphysically, Feminine Genius is Source energy—discarnate Godstuff, a flavor of All That Is—and lives in the "other world" of soul, spirit, mystery, creative energy, and divine intelligence. Physically, Feminine Genius is life-force energy—the flow of life and the power of Creation in each incarnate human body—and lives in "this world" of matter, bodies, battles, feelings, form, and function.

Feminine Genius is an interface between the other world and this world, an interface between you and that which made you. Feminine Genius is an intelligence that you can use to source your life, your choices, and your contributions to the world that is divine in origin and is felt by you in your body.

Feminine Genius is the feminine flavor of God.

WHY "GENIUS"?

The word *genius* almost always evokes an image of Albert Einstein, the Nobel Prize–winning, German-born theoretical physicist, who lived from 1879 to 1955. As famous for his theory of relativity and his mass-energy equivalence formula, $E = mc^2$, as for his shock of wild white hair, many of Einstein's discoveries served as the foundation for modern physics, through quantum theory (which is sexier than it sounds, and I'll share more about in a bit).

We have come to worship Einstein's brain and his intellect, and to assume that great intelligence is *intellectual* intelligence, that great genius is *intellectual* genius. And while it is true that many of Einstein's discoveries were in the intellectual realms of reasons, theories, and ideas, his true genius was in his ability to open not just his reasoning mind but his intuitive mind as well (also known as *soul*). Einstein sported not just intellectual intelligence but intuitive intelligence as well.

Intuitive intelligence comes to us as a set of sensations, emotions, longings, urges, impulses, and images, all felt in the soma, the body. Intuition is less used and less understood as a trusted source of intelligence, partly because it is pre-lingual, meaning that your intuition comes first through your feelings, and then afterward you may be able to put words and meaning to it. Intuition is unruly and vast, rarely literal, and shies away like a wild horse when we try to break it with reasons and rules. Although often hard to understand, wily to work with, and easy to disregard altogether, your intuitive intelligence is no less genius than your intellectual genius. In fact, without it, your life will never be your own.

As Bob Samples writes in his book *The Metaphoric Mind: A Celebration of Creative Consciousness*, "Albert Einstein called the intuitive . . . mind a sacred gift. He added that the rational mind was a faithful servant. It is paradoxical that in the context of modern life we have begun to worship the servant and defile the divine."[1] Although we have positioned Einstein as the model of intellectual genius, he was actually an intuitive, faithful servant of All That Is.

Elizabeth Gilbert, writer, speaker, and champion for the creative fire in us all, sheds further light on our misconceptions about *genius*.

Most of us believe genius is a marking, something like race, economic status, political affiliation, or gender. We believe that either we are a genius—or we are not. But Elizabeth Gilbert shares that for much of history it was understood that genius isn't something you *are*, it is something you *have*—or get visited by. With that understanding, anyone can have a genius, kind of like having a house gnome or kitchen elf. The root of the word *genius* is the same as the word *genie*, after all.

Genius, then, can be re-understood as an unseen but very felt force that enters and operates through us. Genius can be re-understood to be an energy that can animate us and speak through us, and that we can be in deep partnership with. Uncorked, genius helps us, like it helped Einstein, bring enchantment from the other world into this world. Indeed, Einstein parted the veil between this world and the other world, and in flooded the profound, beautiful, and intelligent languages of mathematics and physics. Likewise, when you part the veil between this world and the other world, in floods the profound, beautiful, and intelligent language of Feminine Genius.

FEMININE GENIUS—A LANGUAGE

Any language—whether verbal, somatic, or scientific—is simply a system of communication, a call and response between *what is to be expressed* and *what or who is to express it*. Mathematics and physics, languages used by Einstein, are languages with laws and principles, rules and exceptions, dialects and accents, utterly stunning to behold. They are complete and magnificent languages that have little to do with English (or German, Einstein's first language) but unravel some mysteries about how our miraculous world functions. These languages are at once exact yet also poetic, magical, and often humorous. Some would go so far as to say that gazing at a prime number sequence—or the golden ratio in a nautilus shell, or the power of nuclear fission—is like gazing at God.

Feminine Genius is likewise a language with laws and principles, rules and exceptions, dialects and accents, utterly stunning to behold. It is not about English or German or Afrikaans, yet it unravels for us mysteries about how a woman's world can function most miraculously. It too is a language at once exact, yet also poetic, magical, and often humorous. Some would go so far as to say that gazing at a woman in communion with her body—a woman who is led by her longing and radiant with inner light—is like gazing at God.

I go so far. In fact, I go further.

Feminine Genius is the language itself, and it is also the woman who speaks it. Feminine Genius is intelligence itself, and it is also the woman who knows it.

Einstein's genius was not just his intellect per se, it was what he tapped into and let have its way with his intellect. Yes, he had a strong, playful, curious, and open mind, but his genius was less about how many neurons he had or how deft his gray matter was, and more about the wild and exciting languages he let fully ignite him. Likewise, it is good to cultivate a strong, playful, curious, and open mind (and body, soul, and heart), so Feminine Genius can have its way with you, excite you, and fully ignite you.

And yet, the point of learning the mother tongue of Feminine Genius isn't to get to some point where, at last, you are done expressing yourself. Your blood doesn't stop circulating after one round through your circulatory system, and your brain doesn't stop learning after absorbing one skill. Being fully awake and alive means tapping in continually and deeply to the life-giving, expressive arteries of Feminine Genius.

You don't become a Feminine Genius one day and stay that way, like receiving damehood by the queen of England, and being forevermore a dame. You are always becoming and becoming and becoming. You are always learning and growing. Feminine Genius is a path, not a destination. You are never done. You walk, then you stroll, then you sprint, and then you hold your head up and run the marathon. Feminine Genius needs a lot of enunciation and practice, refinement and repetition, watering and misting and plumping—kind of like a woman does.

As we dive a bit deeper into understanding Feminine Genius, it is worth saying that of course genius works its sorcery through our masculine strengths as well as our feminine strengths. There's nothing inherently wrong with masculine strengths—our rational, linear, go-go-go, get-it-done, goal-oriented, competitive, will-powered abilities. They are needed, they are genius, and they are great. All human beings have within us both masculine and feminine strengths, but we currently overuse our Masculine Genius to the point of personal and cultural breakdown. And, it is my staunch opinion that in order to flourish as a woman in the world today, you need to have your Feminine Genius alive and well, so tended and so watered, in fact, that you are downright juicy, bursting into life.

Before I go into the differences between Masculine and Feminine Genius so that you can use your Feminine Genius as adeptly as you've been taught to use your Masculine Genius, let me take a moment to define some terms.

Gender Can Be Fluid

Masculine, feminine; man, woman; male, female—oh, dear. If ever there were a hornet's nest, this could be one. Yet in I go. As we head into some rather messy but marvelous metaphysical territory, peppered with metaphor and sprinkled with a few scientific theories, I will share what I mean by those terms. I use the terms *masculine* and *feminine* to refer to a quality, energy, or essence. I use the terms *male* and *female* to refer to a physical body with specific gender and sex characteristics. I use the terms *man* and *woman* to refer to the whole and total human being. I leave it up to each person to self-identify as a *man*, or a *woman*, or something else on the spectrum of gender.

Yes, gender is a spectrum. It is good to be clear that gender and sex characteristics are not binary, but rather exist on a continuum. We used to assume that a baby was either a girl or a boy, based on if *she* had a vagina or *he* had a penis. We assumed there were *he*s and *she*s, end of story, and that what showed up on the outside of a body indicated what was inside the body—reproductive organs, brain, temperament, self-expression, and very identity. But in truth, it's all fluid.

In the same way, you don't possess just masculine or just feminine attributes; you have both within you. The world might see you as a man, but you might identify as a woman, or vice versa. And, for example, between two and five people in 1,000 have female sex organs on the outside (like a vulva, vagina, and clitoris) yet have male sex organs on the inside (like testes, a vas deferens, and seminal vesicles). Nature mixes and matches in all kinds of ways. There's no one right way to be. I speak to you, wherever you place yourself on the spectrum of male to female, masculine to feminine, man to woman.

However, it is my belief that you are reading this book because you identify, at least to some degree, as a woman—or at the very least you want to know more about what the heck it takes for a woman to flourish in a world that is built more with men, maleness, and masculine strengths in mind. I assume that you want to learn what Feminine Genius *is*, and how to have a harmonious balance between your Masculine and Feminine Genius.

MASCULINE GENIUS, FEMININE GENIUS

To distinguish Masculine Genius from Feminine Genius, I like this metaphor: Your Masculine Genius is like a locomotive, as in a speedy train. Your Feminine Genius, on the other hand, is more like a cauldron—as in a vessel used by witches and alchemists—in which to combine, heat up, and completely transform potent ingredients. A train travels rapidly from point A to point B, in one direction, toward a goal, steaming ahead. A cauldron stays in one place, more or less, and attracts into it the ingredients it needs, and then gets a nice fire lit under its ass. A train delivers; a cauldron receives. A train transports; a cauldron transforms.

Both trains and cauldrons are useful, but they are not interchangeable. You wouldn't mix them up in your toolbox. Superman, the man of steel, more powerful than a *cauldron*, able to leap buildings in a single bound? I think not. When you need to make a healing salve, intuit your next step, or turn lead into gold, even the most organized, pumped-up, time-managed, and steely locomotive just can't do it.

The ancient symbol of the Divine Masculine is a blade or sword, while the time-honored symbol of the Divine Feminine is the chalice, a sacred vessel and Holy Grail used to hold the elixir of life. Extend the symbology into biology, and you get the sword as penis and the chalice as womb and vagina. The word *vagina* translates literally as "sheath for a sword." While that does drive the point home, so to speak, it is kind of icky. I prefer the vagina and uterus and all a woman's lady parts to be quite definable and useful regardless of whether a sword is or is not present, thank you very much. However, lady parts as sacred vessel? This is a powerful metaphor indeed.

Think about it: a womb doesn't rush out into the wide world to dominate sperm worldwide, only to drag them home by the tails to make a baby. Nope, your sacred chalice sits pretty and magnetizes the potent ingredients she needs to create life itself. You could say that the womb, a metaphoric and literal aspect of Feminine Genius, creates possibility itself from "nothing." Like a cauldron and like a womb, Feminine Genius starts with a fertile void, draws to it what it needs, and creates all shades of life, whether a baby, a book, or a business.

The predominant culture prizes penises, swords, and trains over vaginas, chalices, and cauldrons. I have yet to meet a woman who didn't hold the subconscious fear of fully expressing herself—or of fully *being* herself—whether at the dinner table, at work meetings, or even with friends; a fear of being, figuratively or rather literally, "burned at the stake" for having a cauldron.

Linear Reality, Spiral Reality

Feminine Genius and Masculine Genius, representing two flavors of the Divine, also operate in two different flavors of reality. Masculine Genius operates in what is known as *Newtonian reality*. Sir Isaac Newton lived about four hundred years ago (a few hundred years before Einstein) and is widely recognized as one of the most influential scientists of all time, a key figure in the scientific revolution. A falling apple hit him on the head and led him to an *aha!* moment that changed the course of Western thinking. From that moment, Newton was able to describe the law of gravity and the phenomenon of cause and effect (falling apple and apple hitting head).

In Newtonian reality, time and space are linear and measurable. There are sixty minutes in an hour, and you can use your watch or phone or Big Ben to prove it. Time progresses in one straight line, as evidenced by your birth and your progression toward eventual death. In Newtonian reality, cause comes before effect. Obviously, the falling apple comes before the apple hitting Sir Isaac's head, right? We can see plainly that yesterday happened yesterday, and tomorrow will happen tomorrow.

In Newtonian reality, matter operates in predictable ways. The chair upon which you are now sitting is solid and stable. How could it be otherwise and still hold you up? Objects in the world are separate from each other, and it takes a certain amount of force and energy for one to influence the other, like your hand attempting to grip and lift a barbell.

In Newtonian reality, the body, mind, and soul are seen as separate. Our current views about bodies, minds, and souls are heavily influenced by Newtonian and other related philosophies, like those of René Descartes, a French philosopher, mathematician, and scientist who lived during Newton's lifetime. In Western culture especially, we have inherited the assumptions that the mind is disconnected from the body, and that the body is an inferior vessel whose purpose is to chauffeur the exalted mind through life. We have come to assume that the mind is that which fits inside of and is contained by the skull, and that consciousness itself resides in this localized, contracted mind.

Further influenced by the ideas of many world religions, including Christianity, we tend to believe that divinity is achievable only by leaving the body behind—whether literally when we have died and gone to heaven, or metaphorically when we have completely purified or transcended our unruly, sinful bodies. We assume we exist separate from the Divine, and so live lonely, disconnected lives, believing that our reunion with the Almighty will only happen if we are virtuous enough to make it into "his" favor, into whatever version of heaven we believe in.

However, there is another reality, another possibility. While it is not Newtonian, it is just as significant, and it is what I most want to introduce you to.

Quantum Reality, Divine Reality

While Masculine Genius operates in Newtonian reality, Feminine Genius operates in what is called *quantum* reality. Quantum theory (otherwise known as quantum physics or quantum mechanics) is the basis of modern physics and explains the nature and behavior of matter, light, and energy on the atomic and subatomic levels. Quantum theory has been advanced by folks like Werner Heisenberg, Max Planck, Niels Bohr, and Austrian physicist Erwin Schrödinger, a contemporary of Albert Einstein's, who expanded on Einstein's theory of relativity. Before you start glazing over in the face of quantum theory's fiendish complexity, don't forget that I promised you it is sexy. And it's not just sexy—it's sacred. Allow me to enlighten you.

I think of research into and application of quantum theory as an "emperor wears no clothes" type of scrutiny. Its findings upset the apple cart of conventional reasoning and reality. Said less euphemistically, it revisits established assumptions in science, medicine, and spirituality and comes up with non-linear insights that don't fit what we're used to. For example, whereas the speed of light has been understood as the fastest rate at which anything can travel, quantum theory shows that instantaneous transfer of information seems to be possible. Whereas conventional understanding says that objects separated by great space and time (like you and the moon, or you and your long-distance beloved) can't affect one another, quantum theory shows that there is an invisible stream of energy connecting any two objects so that they will affect one another, forever, regardless of where they are.

Quantum theorists, linking arms with their upstart elder cousins, the Tantrists, find that everything is interconnected, a worldwide web of interdependent life-force energy. Quantum theory reveals that consciousness cannot be confined by our brains. It exists within everything—hence the term *collective consciousness*, a decentralized, yet unified force. In fact, quantum theory has found that our brains, once thought to be like tape recorders, are actually more like TV receivers, receiving and relaying information rather than storing it. Quantum theory redefines an individual mind as collective mind. It is a field of intelligent, powerful, life-force energy that we as human beings arise from and are in constant and direct dialogue with.

Even though quantum theory *begins* by examining the behavior of the tiny particles that make up tiny atoms that make up your arm, your body, a tree, and everything in the universe, quantum theory can *end up* explaining otherwise unexplainable biological and metaphysical phenomena such as the ability to regenerate a limb, to have extrasensory perception (ESP), precognition, telepathy, remote viewing, spontaneous remission, healing, prayer, dream sharing, intuition, and the "collective mind"—or the "collective soul."

I think of quantum theory as the long-awaited merging of two former archenemies: science and the sacred. Quantum theory allows science to explain God, and allows God to communicate with us through science.

Quantum theory not only shows us the "other world" of the far-out and fantastic, it also—by capitalizing on the fascinating behavior of subatomic particles—shows up in "this world" in the everyday wonders of superconducting magnets, light-emitting diodes (LED lights), lasers, transistors, microprocessors, magnetic resonance imaging (MRI machines), and electron microscopy.

Time and Space Can Be Fluid, Too

In quantum reality, in contrast to the linear and measurable world of Newtonian reality, time and space are malleable and fluid. Where Masculine Genius is like a train, busting ass from point A to point B, Feminine Genius is more like a wormhole where time and space bend in on themselves so the distance between point A and point B disappears. Point A spirals and loop-de-loops and curls in intimately toward point B, so that eventually the distance between point A and point B no longer exists, and traveling from point A to point B takes no time at all; it is instantaneous. Where Masculine Genius moves like an arrow, Feminine Genius moves like a slinky.

In quantum reality, as with Feminine Genius, it becomes hard to distinguish effect from cause, since time and space are all wormholed and spiraled in on themselves, so that what comes before what starts to get rather murky. What comes first, the chicken or the egg?

In quantum reality, there is only *now*. In quantum reality, as with Feminine Genius, time is circular, cyclical, and in harmony with All That Is. Today is today, yesterday is today, and tomorrow is also today.

In quantum reality, matter is wily and unpredictable. It turns out that the subatomic particles and molecules that make up the chair upon which you are now sitting—as well as your own body—are actually made up of more open space than actual matter. So your simple act of sitting in a chair is kind of a humorous hallucination because you are actually a patch of nothing perched on a patch of nothing. From "nothing," Feminine Genius is born.

Looking with quantum eyes through the lens of Feminine Genius, you see that you are no longer separate from the Divine; you and the Divine are made of the same stuff. Your mind is not separate from your body, or from your soul; all parts of you are interconnected—and are interconnected with the Holy One. There is nowhere you could go and nothing you could do to fall from the embrace of the Almighty.

Striving, Surfing

Newtonian and quantum realities are both real and true. Both are happening at the same time, just like it is real and true that you have both masculine and feminine essences in you at the same time. Whereas Masculine Genius strives to triumph over (and is often squashed by) space, time, matter, and cause and effect, Feminine Genius strives to surf them.

Masculine Genius operates in *kronos* time (measurable time as you find on a clock or calendar) whereas Feminine Genius operates in *kairos* time—known as "God's time." When you measure time with your Masculine Genius, it will be pretty orderly and predictable, something to manage. When you are using your Feminine Genius, things might go exponentially faster or slower than you are comfortable with.

Masculine Genius is sourced largely from your rational brain, as sensed through your mental reasons, analyses, and judgments.

Feminine Genius is sourced largely from a field of intelligent life-force as felt through your somatic feelings and emotions. You are using your Masculine Genius when you use your *discriminative* mind—analytical and comparative, full of reasons. You are using your Feminine Genius when you tap into your *intuitive* mind—feeling and sensing, connecting the dots.

Your Masculine Genius, adept in Newtonian reality, gathers its information via the single input of here and now. If it were a sound, it would be a simple, catchy melody. Your Feminine Genius, adept in quantum reality, gathers its information via the multiple, simultaneous inputs of your intuition—from all life, from all people, from all sources, from all times, all at once. If it were a sound, it would be a complex, soaring symphony.

Where Feminine Genius parts the veil between this world and the other world, Masculine Genius is busy working to efficiently describe, manufacture, and mass market the veil. Where Masculine Genius is linear, Feminine Genius is cyclical. Where Masculine Genius is constancy, Feminine Genius is change. Where Masculine Genius contains the storm, Feminine Genius *is* the storm.

Where the cauldron of Feminine Genius creates possibility, the train of Masculine Genius makes it manifest. Where Feminine Genius provides the *why*, Masculine Genius provides the *how*. Where Feminine Genius hungers for more, Masculine Genius fulfills the order. When you have an inspired desire to create something, that is your Feminine Genius at play. When you are ass kicking, name taking, and making it happen, that's your Masculine Genius. When your Masculine Genius sets goals, gets productive, and handles deadlines—and when it does so in faithful service to your deepest desires—I like to say that it is a faithful servant to your Feminine Genius, which turns out to be a truly aligned and balanced way to be, work, and walk through life.

A FEMININE GENIUS WAY OF BEING

> If we are in constant and instantaneous dialogue
> with our environment, if all the information from
> the cosmos flows through our pores at every
> moment, then our current notion of our human
> potential is only a glimmer of what it could be.
>
> LYNNE McTAGGART, *The Field: The Quest for the Secret Force of the Universe*

Feminine Genius is not just a type of person, it is also a way of being. Or actually, it is a vein of energy, a force of love and light that, if you tap it, will without hesitation flood through your body and life, informing your desires, shaping your visions, and guiding you to real, honest-to-goodness, everyday fulfillment. At the end of the day, you are answering one important question with your life: in what ways does the Divine wish to live *as* you and *through* you? Your Masculine Genius's job is to help get your answers out into the world. But the answers—your answers—are best spoken with the language of your Feminine Genius.

So, again, Feminine Genius is the intelligence that you use to source your life, your choices, and your contribution to the world that is divine in origin and felt by you in your body.

Oh, fellow Feminine Genius, I know what you hunger for.

Of course we are all unique. Like snowflakes, no two women are the same. Yet your woman's heart is like mine, is like the hearts of my clients, readers, course participants, friends, and family. You long to feel in deep partnership with All That Is—that which made you. To feel sensuously, unabashedly, and utterly comfortable in your own skin. To share your light, without burning out.

To know that you are not too much—but that you are enough, more than enough. That you are not and never were damaged goods. That there is nothing, and I mean nothing, inside you or about you to be ashamed of. There never was.

And that your shame is also beautiful.

Whether man, woman, or something more fluid, the Divine is having one heck of a human experience, *through* you and *as* you. How you animate her, give her voice, wings, legs, a pen, a paintbrush, or a heart, is up to you.

It is not wrong that you long. Your hunger is holy. You are the holder of a vision for a better, brighter world (or office, family, community, or piece of art) that's not quite here yet, and needs to be. Your passion makes you ache. Do not attempt to fix, fade, solve, absolve, or medicate the ache. Ache is a preferred dialect of Feminine Genius.

Feminine Genius asks you to adore your ache and to ride it like a magic carpet, and find your way home. Feminine Genius asks you to use your aching, intuitive, intelligent body to bring enchantment from the other world into this world, and remake the whole wide world into one that works for everyone.

Feminine Genius is the One who said, "Let there be light," and is also the woman who, even through the darkest of nights, continues walking into her bright life.

Will you go there with me now?

> The place you are right now,
> God circled on a map for you.
> **HAFIZ**

Part Two

Navigating Your Dark

5

Dying To Live
All Great Journeys Begin in the Dark

For a seed to achieve its greatest expression,
it must come completely undone. The shell cracks,
its insides come out and everything changes.
To someone who doesn't understand growth,
it would look like complete destruction.
CYNTHIA OCCELLI

When I was pregnant—and at the beginning of my journey of creating new human life—I spent months researching and practicing to have a natural birth at home, and ideally one that would be pleasurable. So often, women's expectations for childbirth are limited to scary, freaky, and painful with a side of anesthesia. So I thought, why not imagine—and potentially experience—something wonderful instead?

I listened to over thirty lectures by midwives, doctors, doulas, researchers, and mothers. I danced, did yoga, took naps, and because I was also supposed to have lots of sex and lots of orgasms, my husband was happy to get seriously involved. It just made sense: I had been studying and practicing how to make my life more pleasurable for years, and it was a theme in my coaching practice as well.

And yet, at the same time that I practiced like an Olympian for a pleasurable birth, I became more aware of death. It wasn't just that I was aware that I could die in childbirth, or that I might be entirely unequipped to keep my tiny wisp of a baby alive. It was also as if I had been playing in the sunshine all my life and suddenly noticed that there were shadows everywhere—and I could not take my eyes off them. The dark aspect of all things whispered to me. I couldn't make out what it was saying exactly, but it sounded important, vital, and badass. I did feel a little weird to be so *noire* at a time that was all about tender new life, but I was fascinated. Interested. Willing. This kind of death didn't feel like the opposite of life, but more like life's long-lost twin.

When I went into labor, I was ready. I put all my pleasure strategies to use. I breathed, stretched, kissed my husband, did lunges down the hall, squatted, got in the shower, lowed like a cow, got out of the shower, got in the birth tub, talked with the baby, visualized my womb opening like a lotus flower, got out of the birth tub, kissed my husband, and did more lunges down the hall.

After trying for twenty hours to turn the pain of labor into sensations of pleasure, I internally gave the finger to my home birth teacher who had said contractions lasted for about a minute. Mine were easily two minutes with very little rest in between. I retreated into another realm where I couldn't even remember the word *pleasure*. I was in agony. I closed my eyes and listened for guidance. *There's no way out for him*, my inner voice said, referring to my baby. And then I sensed a series of images: the front door of my house opening into the front door of the hospital, opening into the door of the operating room: C-section.

WTF? Okay, first of all, "no way out"? Of course there's a way out. It is called giving birth. All babies have a way out. It is called my vagina, thank you very much. Vaginas happen to be really, really good at getting babies out into the world. And this labor-induced vision, that is the opposite of what I planned for? I don't think so. No. No, thank you.

I did more lunges. More lowing. For another two hours.

Then my midwife checked again on my dilation and the baby's position. With a worried cast to her eyes, she whispered to her partner, "Transverse arrest." They exchanged a foreboding look. "Get her overnight bag, and we'll meet you at the hospital," they said to my husband. Just like that, my pleasure plan evaporated. Exhausted and dehydrated, I threw pleasure under the bus and prayed fervently for narcotics. I literally wept as the drugs were injected into my body, and I could finally see again. With my baby's heartbeat slowing alarmingly, they wheeled me into the operating room.

My baby was born healthy and beautiful (well, more like cute old man alien) with all his fingers and all his toes intact. The doctor who performed the C-section—who looked like one of the gorgeous blonde interns from the TV show *Grey's Anatomy*—said she had never had to pull so hard to get a baby out. Either he or I would have likely died without her intervention.

"Sometimes a blessing comes in the form of a scalpel," my friend Sera told me. But I couldn't yet see the C-section as a godsend. It felt like a curse for failing my god of pleasure.

As I nursed my newborn, I read about transverse arrest and discovered why it is so alarming: instead of coming out crown-of-head first, the baby tries to come out side-of-head first and gets stopped, too big to pass through mom's pelvic opening. In medical texts, transverse arrest is a rare and dangerous complication, known as the "no way out" position.

No way out. I started to cry. And then to laugh. I hadn't thought to share my strange birth vision with my midwife. I thought it was nonsense or fear rather than wisdom and premonition. Because I was *expecting* a vision of my vagina opening as a sacred flower, letting my baby slip ecstatically into this world, I ignored my *actual* and alarming vision of the doors opening to operating tables and scalpels, the doctors prying my baby out of my body. I cried and laughed some more, unsettled by the eerie power of my inner voice and vision.

Still, even with this understanding, it took me nearly two years to completely unravel my shame at my birth gone crosswise. I agonized over what I had missed. How had I been so unable to make the birth pleasurable? I was supposed to be the expert. Many of my friends labored for thirty, forty, even fifty hours and in the end had natural births. I was trained as a dancer to perform through any catastrophe, even a broken toe. (I have, in fact, performed once or twice with a broken toe.) How could my training and resolve have crumbled so completely? My plan had failed. I had failed my plan. My plan had failed because I was a failure. If I hadn't turned into such a *fake*, I thought, perhaps I could have had my kiddo at home and avoided ingesting more painkillers in a few hours than I had in my entire lifetime. For what was I being punished?

It took time to understand that not getting what I wanted or had prepared for so diligently was actually a blessing. I reviewed the facts and let them shed light on the fog of my shame. Slowly, slowly, I realized that if the birth had gone according to *my* plan, I would have assumed that any outcome I wanted was always in my control. I would have assumed that my plan was the best plan. I would have assumed, a bit smugly, that any pain can be transmuted into pleasure. But the truth is, some kinds of pain can be transmuted and other kinds simply fucking hurt.

If the birth had gone according to plan, I would have continued to feel a tiny bit separate from and elevated over other women and mothers, those poor, lazy suckers who didn't get what they labored for. "I've made a plan; I've done my research; I've followed my plan; and therefore, I deserve a great result," would have remained my thinking. I would have smiled compassionately on others' heartbreaks, feeling safe and secure on my high horse.

I would have continued to believe, as I learned from the worlds of dance, media, and culture, that mothering, parenting, creating, working, or simply being alive and a woman, is a competition. Which is life stealing.

I would have continued to attach my worth as a human being to any outcome I planned for and worked toward. Which is toxic.

I would have continued to dismiss the voice inside me that knew exactly what the hell it was talking about, and I would have missed learning the markings of intuition that distinguish the voice of inner knowing from the voice of fear. Which is tragic.

Don't get me wrong, I like getting what I want. Sometimes I hit it out of the park, and it feels good. And I am also overjoyed for the women who have given birth on their own terms, even pleasurably. I no longer take one woman's triumph to mean my defeat. But now

I also know that getting what I want is no longer the main event. Which is what the dark death aspect of my pregnancy had come to teach me. As it turns out, all great journeys begin in the dark.

In our shadow—that dark underworld of our psyche that holds all we have disowned, aren't ready to see, cannot yet feel, or refuse to look at—nestles a seed germinating a new part of ourselves. The day I birthed my baby, I also birthed a new part of myself. My baby's birthday will forevermore also be *my* birthday. And for another part of me, it will also be my death-day. The blessings of the dark hold true for literal and figurative mothers alike. Blessings, all, from the divine offices of Feminine Genius herself. Oh, hello, darkness, our old friend.

INVITATION TO THE DARK

The complete destruction of a plan, the alchemical burning of out-worn parts of yourself, or the unadorned heartbreak that brings you to your knees are simply your invitations to descend into the dark, into the bright holy death part of the cycle of death and rebirth.

The dark requires you to compost your rotten ideas about yourself and create fertile soil from which you can burst into life. The dark asks you to renounce your false idols of "getting it right," to renovate the shrine to your intuitive voice, and to resurrect the belief that blessings often come in wolf's clothing. (Scalpel, anyone?)

The dark outlines your heart with indelible black marker so that whatever was previously invisible, you can now see in stark relief. The dark reminds you that you are not being punished; you are being *invited*. The dark reminds you that feeling, "I can't. No really, I am not kidding; I truly don't have it in me," is a sure sign that you are about to do the impossible—although not in the way you planned to do it, of course.

Feminine Genius, this patron saint of women worldwide, has plans for you, too. She prefers curveballs to remove separation between you and other women, between warring parts of yourself, and between you and the Divine. She is a straight shooter, helping you hone your inner wisdom and your courage to follow it. She is a righteous badass who favors tough love, yet knows when to apply the balm of grace. She brandishes both dark and light, whatever it takes to kill your illusions and bring you more to life. Absolute genius, she prefers to wear your face in the mirror. Girl, Feminine Genius looks good on you.

With all due respect to the different forms and degrees of our dark times, all women need to learn black-belt-level skills so we can navigate the dark, whatever dark may come our way, whether from the big mama in the cosmos or the big daddy of our dominant culture. Because there is something more important than getting what we wanted with our whole hearts. More important than any plan is all that we must learn and unlearn, and the woman we must grow into as we do.

"Easy for you to say," you might reply. "In the end, your baby was healthy and so were you. Easy to find a lesson and a blessing in that. Explain to me, if you can, why *that* woman's baby died, why *that* woman can't have a baby at all despite spending a small fortune in fertility treatments, why *that* woman's sister got hit by a bus, why *her* country is torn apart by genocide, why *she* is dying of bone cancer, why *she* had acid thrown in her face, why *she* was raped and left for dead, why *she* was passed over for the promotion."

There's no way to explain pain and heartbreak, no way to measure blessing and grace. This isn't a competition. Mine isn't better or worse than yours. Trying to measure is madness. Trying to explain is beside the point. Plus, you can't hear your inner truth if you are too high up on your high horse.

> Rupture is not where your story ends.
> It is where it begins.
> **REGENA THOMASHAUER**

So, one day, as you are shooting for the moon and landing among the stars, Feminine Genius will divert your itinerary and hurl you into the underworld. "WTF? What just happened? Where the hell am I?" you will likely ask.

"Come on down from that horse," she will say. "Come on in. And don't mess around swimming in circles in the shallow end. Dive deep.

Descend. That's right, let's go down. All the way down. Come on in," she will invite you with a toothy grin, "the water's fine."

I can't. This is impossible. Will this ever end? I can't do it. I can't make it through. It's too much. It's too long. I thought I dealt with this already. This is impossible. It will never end. This is what you will think when you are down in the dark and everything has been invaded with the chill of your personal wintertime. It *will* be too much. It *will* be too long. You *will* have dealt with this already. It *will* be impossible. It *will* never end.

And then it will end.

> Sometimes when you're in a dark place you think you've been buried but you've actually been planted.
> **CHRISTINE CAINE**

6

Living with Your Cycles
The Journey from Death to Rebirth

We don't receive wisdom; we must discover
it for ourselves after a journey that no one
can take for us or spare us.

MARCEL PROUST, *In Search of Lost Time*

Nature loves her cycles. And those cycles naturally include a good spell of darkness. Nature includes darkness, shadow, and death in her grand design of life. Nature adores a good death as much as a good rebirth.

Nature builds things up, makes them bloom into stunning beauty, then strips them bare, sends them into stasis, and piles on snow, sleet, and ice. And then she does it all over again. Forever, there have been winters and summers, deaths and rebirths—rinse and repeat. Why should it be any different for us humans? We are part of the natural world, after all.

So then, it would seem that the point of your life isn't to try and get all your physical, financial, and spiritual ducks in a row so you can stay in the eternal sunshine of summer. It is also to repeatedly get thrust into dark, mysterious winters. Because as you align with nature's cycles, you also align with the intelligence of the natural world. You feel less crazy, flawed, and separate, and you feel more like a sacred strand of the whole web of life.

As my C-section scars slowly healed, and I shrugged off my shroud of shame, I began to wonder if *everything* has an intelligent and artful design, even the mythic plagues of locusts and the re-routed birth stories. If we are meant to be in winter as much as in summer, in challenge as much as in celebration, then mustn't there be profound wisdom within every wintry breakdown—and within the cycle itself?

There is.

But as a woman living in the modern age and relying too much on your Masculine Genius—your rational, linear, go-go-go, get-it-done, goal-oriented, competitive, will-powered abilities—it is likely that you, like too many of us, are sorely disconnected from nature and from the cyclical nature of your body, mind, and soul. In the Western world—even here where women have unprecedented free-doms, rights, opportunities, and equalities (hallelujah!)—the models for success and leadership are largely masculine. So your attempts to live, work, work out, earn money, eat, sleep, decide, meditate, have sex, and generally be fulfilled are usually driven by your Masculine Genius overpowering your Feminine Genius. In a "man's world," it is all too easy to turn away from the seasons of death and rebirth that make the natural world—and the world inside of you—go round.

Why shouldn't every summertime come to a close, giving each of us a breather, allowing us to harvest, and then to compost? Why do we want to live forever in never-ending triumph? Why do we resist slowing down, shedding skin, and sowing seeds for our next jubilant springtime? Where is the training manual—heck, the honorary degree—for lying fallow?

Who are we to think we could—and *should*—escape the cycles of the natural world? Who are we to think that we are somehow separate from the natural world? Or that it is more spiritual to transcend, more virtuous to vanquish the natural world? Who are we to live so arrogantly? Miserable, that's who.

So then, what if you knew, marrow deep, that you were never meant to always go-go-go, but instead to ebb and flow? What if you knew that the times when you are caught in pain and doubt, like endless dark winters, do not mark the end of your story but rather an auspicious beginning? What if you knew that going through a bad time could be a good thing? Would you feel less broken? Less batty? Would you start to feel more like a hero and less like a victim? Or more like a heroine, I should say, a courageous and wise heroine, honing your courage and wisdom chops on your Heroine's Journey?

FROM THE HERO'S JOURNEY TO THE HEROINE'S JOURNEY

As you may know, a courageous and wise American mythologist named Joseph Campbell studied people's stories across cultures and over time. He noticed their commonalities, and mapped them into a few general recurring storylines. Somewhat condensed, they are: the call to adventure; refusal of the call; crossing the threshold into the abyss of death and rebirth; tests, enemies, and allies; the revelation; and return home with the elixir. All in all, these myths comprise something we know as the *Hero's Journey*, a term Campbell also coined.

Culturally, the Hero's Journey has helped many of us embrace wickedly scary experiences such as falling, failing, feeling lost, and going down into the unknown. The Hero's Journey has repositioned the experience of being faced with insurmountable obstacles from a mistake to a necessary and noble part of *any* meaningful journey. Moviemakers (think Disney, Pixar, and George Lucas), who tell their stories on IMAX screens and in hi def, model their storylines on the Hero's Journey because it hits us all right in our archetypal gut. We nod, and our ancestors nod along with us. We recognize the story because it is part of our story. For our linear, goal-oriented culture of achievement junkies, Campbell's formulation helps us reconnect to the primal idea of the journey and the cycle.

And yet.

Joseph Campbell was a *man*, studying stories and myths largely retold *by* men, largely about the journeys *of men*, at a time when (white) men's experience was considered to be the experience of all humans. Most of our history has been recorded and retold by men, purposely or accidentally leaving out the women. Most of the Hero's

Journey is the *human* journey and isn't gender specific, but some of it actually is quite specific to the *hero* as defined and lived in the form of the Masculine Genius.

In my view, the main difference between the Hero's and Heroine's Journey is this: in a Hero's Journey, the enemies to be vanquished, the mentors to lend a hand, and the guardians to schmooze, the elixir to return home with, all remain separate from and "other" from the hero. In the Heroine's Journey, which is more of a spiral than a straight line, all players, enemies and helpers alike, are internalized in the heroine herself. They are all parts of her.

This is somewhat similar to Jungian dream analysis. My longtime friend Alex, daughter of a clinical psychologist, once told me that, through the Jungian lens, I could choose to view all the characters in my nightly dreams as if they were actually parts of myself. Like Jungian analysts, I needn't see them as actual characters in my external life, but instead as a re-enactment of a struggle—and then a reconciliation—between the parts of me as a whole. That perspective helped me look at my nighttime dreams as journeys within myself, every role played by me. For me, this was an eye-opening perspective, one I have found as invaluable in dreamtime as in waking life.

If all the players in your life journey are recast as aspects of yourself, then the distinction between victim and perpetrator, between enemy and hero, between victor and vanquished, must (or should) dissolve. The inherent setup of enemy = bad, hero = good; perpetrator = guilty, victim = innocent; victor = virtuous, vanquished = poor, miserable slob, dissolves also. As a heroine, you realize that it's all you, and that it's all *within* you, and by trying to defeat an enemy, you are only defeating a part of yourself.

When you are at war with yourself and you win, as my mentor said, who loses? As a heroine both in the external world and in your internal world, you cannot cut out any one part without damaging the whole. You cannot call another the enemy without becoming a victim. You cannot slay an adversary without dishonoring yourself. So as a heroine, you lay down your weapons, realizing you were only going to cut off your own arm anyway.

A brilliant quality of Feminine Genius is interconnectivity: the quantum-inspired, Tantra-inspired understanding that all parts of life are conjoined and intimately related. Where the hero learns to triumph over his obstacles, the heroine learns to open to her obstacles—so they may break her heart open. While the hero may have to burn down his challenges, the heroine invites her challenges to alchemically burn away any untruth within her. Where the hero fights to keep his doubts at a safe distance, the heroine invites her doubts to penetrate her very soul. A hero declares, "I must *ignore* all painful feelings so that I can do this thing I don't feel like doing." A heroine declares, "I must *feel* every painful feeling fully while I do this thing I don't feel like doing."

A hero's mission is to win the battle, but the heroine's mission is to announce that, funny enough, the battle has gone AWOL. The hero wins by defeating the enemy; the heroine wins by declining to perceive a war at all. Where the hero learns new ways to slay his demons, the heroine learns that every demon, when seen rightly, is a friend; and the voice of that friend is her inner voice. The hero takes his journey and finds his way home; the heroine takes her journey and finds that she herself *is* home.

As I see it, the heroine who views her journey through this radical lens of the Heroine's Journey *becomes* a Feminine Genius.

But no matter what, it seems that heroes as well as heroines, Masculine as well as Feminine Geniuses, must be tested. Something courageous and wise within you is invited to rise to the occasion of a challenge. Often, to take your tests and meet your challenges, you must go into the dark, into the unknown, into your shadow. I use the term *shadow* as Carl Jung himself did, to mean an aspect of your psyche that contains the parts of yourself that you have repressed, resisted, disowned, shamed, despised, or simply have yet to meet.

At first whiff, the shadow can seem dangerous and ominous. It is, after all, the unknown, which often feels equated with death. But I see the shadow as the domain of the hilarious as much as the harrowing. Ancient Vedic Tantric philosophy sees existence as playful, downright cheeky in fact, playing a cosmic game of hide-and-seek with us, even as we quake in our Feminine Genius boots. *Leela*, a Sanskrit word that means "the divine play of life," must have a good play with us now and then. We humans are tragically funny after all.

One of your challenges as a Feminine Genius is to walk right into your shadow, to say *yes* to playing the game of life (and death), and to willingly seek that which has been hidden from you. And to be willing for a part of yourself to die. The cycle of being a woman includes the shadow, just like the cycle of the natural world includes the wintertime. For women and nature alike, I call this the death/rebirth cycle.

Just like the wintertime strips a tree of its leaves, the dark strips you of your emotional clothing. Leela, with that distinctively dark sense of humor, lays you bare and deprives you of your familiar tools, landmarks, and abilities. She then smacks your ass and pushes you into the death part of the death/rebirth cycle, trusting that you will see again what you once resisted, that you will meet again what you once disavowed, and that you will embrace again what you once shamed. Leela wants you to have a sacred homecoming, to become a wiser, more courageous version of your precious self. She wants you to have the holy, holy joy of discovering that you had it in you all along.

> What you resist, persists.
> **CARL JUNG**

And, as you might suspect by now, Leela's other name is Feminine Genius. The Heroine's Journey's other name is the path of Feminine Genius. And we cannot take even one single step on the path of Feminine Genius without treading on the death/rebirth cycle.

Feelings of *ugly*, *flawed*, *failed*, and *forsaken*—all markers of the death part of the death/rebirth cycle—are generally extremely painful. Yet, you suffer less from the pain, and more because you view death in any form as a period in your sentence, rather than a comma. You assume failure marks the *end* of a journey, when really it marks the *beginning*. When you have no real understanding of what the death parts of the death/rebirth cycle are truly about, it is not only unfortunate, it is also crazy making.

I once heard the saying, "An old sailor is one who has learned to respect the sea." And so it is in this understanding of the word *respect* that I say that every woman must learn to deeply respect the death/rebirth cycle—or resign to feeling tossed about on an infinite ocean of insanity, uncertainty, doubt, and disease. A Feminine Genius, then, learns to truly live with the death/rebirth cycle.

every moment is either a challenge or a celebration, a death or a rebirth

THE DEATH/REBIRTH CYCLE IN ITS MANY EXPRESSIONS

An obvious place to see the death/rebirth cycle at work is in the seasons of the natural world: winter, spring, summer, and fall. True, not all parts of the world have four distinct seasons, yet all parts of the world have seasonal cycles, even if they are subtle, that fluctuate between wetter and drier, or hotter and cooler.

In the death/rebirth cycle, fall and winter (or the cooler, wetter seasons) are times of death, where things fall away and are harvested, characterized by darkness, coolness, cold, challenge, stillness, and dormancy. Physically and metaphysically, fall and winter are times to receive and release. Metaphysically, the death part of the death/rebirth cycle is the *unknown*.

In the death/rebirth cycle, spring and summer (or hotter, drier seasons) are times of rebirth, where things sprout and bloom, characterized by light, warmth, heat, celebration, movement, and growth. Physically and metaphysically, spring and summer are times to renew and rejoice. Metaphysically, the rebirth part of the death/rebirth cycle is the *known*.

While you might prefer one season to another, you are not likely to condemn the natural world for its cyclic rhythm. In nature, we can see an intelligent force at work that creates and sustains life itself. Fall and winter always come, at first ripe with change, before they turn chill, seemingly interminable, and stark. And then, spring and summer always come, at first bright with possibility, and then hot, persistent, and lovely. What you don't doubt in nature, you could do well to revere in yourself.

again and again, out of each dark winter you will bloom into your own personal springtime

The Seasonality of Your Hormones

Another obvious place to see the death/rebirth cycle at work is in the seasonality of your hormones. I first learned of this concept from my friend and colleague Alisa Vitti, author of *WomanCode*, whom I met and fell in sister love with during my coach training program. One hot summer evening, I sat in Alisa's tiny studio apartment in Hell's Kitchen in New York City as she explained to me how the four weeks of a menstrual cycle correspond to the four seasons in nature, as well as the protocols she was developing at her "FLO Living" center for hormonal healing, including "period tracking," "cycle synching," and "embodied time management," to help any woman flourish by working with her menstrual fluctuations.

Are you crazy? I thought to myself. *Any woman knows that to get ahead, you have to work around your menstrual cycle, not with it.* But that was the last time I thought Alisa—and the genius of the feminine cycle—was crazy. Now, I'm a practicing, somewhat zealous, convert. Allow me to share more about the wisdom that Alisa tapped into and helped me—and countless other lucky women—tap into.

In the female body, hormones are designed to help your moods, emotions, arousal, energy, and focus *fluctuate*. Like a slinky. In the male body, hormones are designed to help the male's moods, emotions, arousal, energy, and focus *regulate*. Like a straight arrow. The female body cycles partly to become fertile, pregnant, and to gestate new life, and an obvious sign of this fertility cycle is menstruation. However, even if you are not menstruating at this time in your life, or you are open only to gestating new ideas rather than gestating new babies, your hormones will still bring you up, down, and all around.

If you menstruate regularly, the death/rebirth cycle will show up pretty much monthly through spiraling fluctuations in your moods, emotions, arousal, energy, and focus, along with obvious physical markers like several days of menstrual bleeding. If you are not currently menstruating, the death/rebirth cycle will still show up pretty much the same way, with the monthly fluctuations in your moods, emotions, arousal, energy, and focus—minus the bleeding.

Now, check out this synchronicity between nature's cycles and women's cycles. The average woman's fertility cycle is around twenty-eight days long, the same length of time the moon goes through her phases. In roughly four weeks, about the time it takes for the moon to cycle from new moon to waxing moon to full moon to waning moon, a menstruating woman's body moves from menstruation phase (bleeding) to the follicular phase (building up the lining of the uterus) to ovulation (fertile, impregnate-able) to the luteal phase (premenstruation, shedding the lining of the womb).

In fact, for some women—especially those who use very few artificial light sources and electrified devices like cell phones, TVs, tablets, and computers—their menstrual cycles map quite elegantly to the cycles of the moon. They bleed during the week of the dark, no-moon; they build up the lining of their uterus during the week of the waxing, building-up moon; they ovulate—meaning, they release a full, ripe egg into their now-fertile womb—during the full, ripe moon; and they begin the process of shedding the lining of their uterus during the waning moon, beginning its descent into the dark again. In my Northern California neck of the woods, many women affectionately call their menstrual cycle their "moon." In true quantum fashion, the moon and your body are in fact interconnected.

By the way, if your menstrual cycle doesn't follow the phases of the moon (mine doesn't), or if it isn't a nice, neat twenty-eight days (mine isn't), don't worry. Menstrual cycle lengths and qualities are as varied as are women, and some women don't menstruate at all or for periods of time (so to speak). However, unless you are in menopause, no longer have a uterus, or are on medication to cease or regulate your cycles, not menstruating (or experiencing pain and life-disruption during menstruation) can mean that something is off in your biochemistry. (For my recommended resources to support your healthy cycling, including Alisa's app for Cycle Synching™ and tools for Period Typing and Embodied Time Management, visit liyanasilver.com/bookresources.)

Think about this for a good hard minute. The same cosmic intelligence that escorts the moon through her phases also ushers in and out the tides of the ocean, and also orchestrates the fluctuations in your human female body. Wow, huh? Like the moon, yours is a celestial body. You couldn't escape the cosmic intelligence of nature if you tried, although we certainly do try.

When my mentee Katya—who you will meet in part three—was seriously underweight at the height of her anorexia, she stopped menstruating for over two years. Although she knew that might be problematic, she didn't care. She was relieved to have removed one more piece of evidence that her body was female. She was eager to continue contorting her woman's body into that of an adolescent boy's body, the ideal in many styles of fashion and media. The shame about fertility runs rampant, whether it's around menstruating "too early" in your life, or "too late," or—as in Katya's case—not menstruating at all. For so many women, there is shame around being unable to become pregnant when you want to, as well as around leaving the childbearing years behind and entering perimenopause and menopause.

But this stigma covers up a potent secret: *that* you cycle means you can create, as God herself creates, whether you are creating a tiny human, composing a rambling poem, or drafting new legislation. Menstruating or not, you cycle. And that you cycle means you can know what God herself knows—the secret of creation. It turns out that your cycle isn't a messy inconvenience after all. It is bright red proof that the intelligence that runs the entire universe also runs through your feminine form.

Ready for even more fascinating symmetry? As Alisa shared with me, our hormonal fluctuations can be figuratively mapped onto the *qualities,* or "moods," that the four seasons of the natural world evoke. When your energy slows, and you feel like hibernating and visioning (often during the bleeding phase, if you are menstruating), it can feel as though you are in a personal *wintertime.* When your energy starts to increase, and you feel adventurous and clever (often during the follicular phase where you are building up the lining of your uterus, if you are menstruating), it can feel as though you are in a personal *springtime.* When your energy abounds, and you feel bold, highly creative, and hot to trot (often during the ovulatory phase, if you are menstruating), it can feel as though you are in a personal *summertime.* And when your energy wanes, and you introspect and harvest your learning (often during the luteal phase, if you are menstruating), it can feel as though you are in a personal *fall.* Beautifully aligned is what you are, in your natural state. And when you are aligned in this way, it is, as Alisa writes, "when you'll feel the fullness of your power, your life-force energy, and your fullest potential."[1]

Emotional and Erotic Fluctuations

It is likely that you will feel distinct emotions during each phase of the death/rebirth cycle. As your hormonal fluctuations bring you into a fall and winter (or death) time, you can experience rage, grief, depression, apathy, doubt, sadness, shame, resentment, anxiety, and blame. As you fluctuate into a spring and summer (or rebirth) time, you can experience joy, gratitude, celebration, happiness, satiation, pride, and confidence. Even more than this, each emotion goes through its own death and rebirth cycle. Whether it is rage or joy or anything in between, each emotion follows the cycle, creeping up or exploding on the scene, building in stormy crescendos, then ebbing, and eventually coming to completion.

The same is true of sexual desire: it cycles. Yearning and waiting can feel wintry; arousal and anticipation can feel spring-like; climax and fulfillment can feel summer-hot; and satisfaction and afterglow can feel autumnal. In French, the expression for orgasm is *la petite mort*, "the little death." It is likely that the types of erotic fantasies you have, the quality of touch you crave, and the speed of lovemaking that feels right to you will shift dramatically as you cycle. Sinking into this understanding can be quite a relief if you have tried, like so many women have, to alter your eroticism to be more like a man's (or like an imagined ideal) and have assumed yourself to be shameful, insufficient, or problematic as a result.

Simply knowing that your desires and emotions are designed to ebb and flow, to come and to go, may help relieve you of some shame and constriction around your feelings, body, and longings. Aligning with your cycles won't inoculate you against the ups and downs, but it does make them feel more natural and workable. In the coming chapters, I'll invite you to artfully work with both your emotions and your erotic energy. I'll invite you to see them not just as hormonal storms to be endured or ignored, or devious forces to be resisted or regretted, but as wise messengers from—and fortifiers of—your soul.

TRULY LIVING WITH YOUR CYCLES

The death/rebirth cycle—the epic and ongoing voyage of Feminine Genius—is not linear; it's helical. It's not straight; it's curvaceous. You can go through the physical and metaphysical death/rebirth cycle in a single day, a single week, or over a whole year. In some cases, the cycle sprawls mysteriously over decades. At any given moment, you are in one part of the death/rebirth cycle or another, in an actual or metaphoric fall, winter, spring, or summer, constantly cycling.

As you cycle between death and rebirth, you cycle between the unknown and the known, down and up, dark and light, rupture and repair, falling and rising, going within yourself and going out into the world, failing and triumphing. When you descend into the dark, you enter into the inner world, the other world: you introspect, you dream, you guess, you disintegrate, and then you grope to find and reassemble the lost parts of yourself. When you ascend into the light, you swagger into the outer world, this world: you take sure-footed actions, you speak, you manifest, you know your truth, and then you speak your truth and give your gifts to the world.

While it is powerful to decline to feel disgraced by your ups and downs, it is even more powerful to adjust to living with your cycles rather than wishing them away, to slow down and sync up instead of driving forward at any cost. Marina, a yoga teacher and health coach (also part wood nymph, I think), joined my mentorship program a couple of years back. She told me that the greatest lesson she learned from aligning with her cycles was how to balance out her natural drive toward productivity and perfection, achievement and success.

As she puts it, "Overscheduling, overworking, and overbooking was a pattern I had for what seems like thirty years. All those years, I learned how not to feel—how to numb, how to retract, how to hide, how to not need help, even from my husband. I now know how powerful it is to have abundance of space in my day and my week so that I can meditate and connect with my wisdom, lean into pleasure, lean into my senses—you know, stop and smell the roses. There is a richness here, a magic." Syncing with your cycles takes courage. And vulnerability. While Marina believes it's the real way to love and connection, it can also bring up the things that were being covered up in the first place.

But courage is native to Feminine Genius. Whereas Marina and her husband used to fight several times a week and well into the night, disrupting their normal, daily rhythms, they rarely fight anymore. They both desperately wanted to connect more and fought as a way to engage. But now, as she has softened, so has he. As she has found a way to express herself and her wants, desires, and needs —which she could only do with enough time and space to connect with herself and hear her own voice—he has found a way to meet her. Where Marina's work used to feel like a *have to* it now feels like a *get to*, and she feels a greater sense of ease, inspiration, and enjoyment in her everyday life. Instead of just making it through, she feels like she is truly living.

> We remember that the user's manual we picked up
> on the way to this planet is in our guts.
> **TASHA BLACK**

Secretly or overtly, you might, as most of us do, prefer times of rebirth. Who doesn't long for more light and more heat in the summertime of their soul, more rejoicing and feeling like a million bucks? Secretly or overtly, you might feel, as most of us do, frankly terrified of times of death and darkness in the wintertime of your soul. The dark can be hard and scary, but is made harder and scarier when we resist it. As a culture, we pathologize and medicate the death part of the death/rebirth cycle, partly because we think it means we will really die. As a culture, we fear slowing down because we think it means we will stop. We forget, collectively, that there is a time to plant things and let them germinate, just like there is a time to harvest them and enjoy their bloom. You might, like most of us do, want to be *on* all the time, feel confident all the time, and be outward bound *all the time*, but that prejudice is killing you.

You think that there is no time for falling or failing, or cycling or ebbing, that you must bring your A game at all times. But really, falling, or failing, is part of the grand plan. As is rising. Falling isn't a misstep; it is a deliberate stepping-stone on the path of Feminine Genius. The part of you that falls is not the same part of you that rises. And only in the depths of your fall will you meet or discover or assemble anew that part of you who will rise.

So go discover how the death/rebirth cycle is cycling in you.

CYCLES PRACTICE   **TRACK IT**

First, each day for at least a month, begin by recording the following three things. Ideally, you will do this recording at the end of your day:

1 Your predominant emotions that day.
2 Your predominant energy level that day.
3 Your predominant beliefs (or thoughts) that day.

Do this every day for at least one month, ideally three, so you can start to see the pattern of your daily emotions, energy, and beliefs.

Especially if you are menstruating regularly—but even if you aren't—the month will likely start to form into two distinct stages of the death/rebirth cycle.

- **Death, or fall/winter,** when your emotions will likely be more tender, introspective, judgmental, and self-effacing. This is when your energy will likely be more inward, slow, deliberate, and thick; and where your thoughts will likely be marked by questioning, doubting, dot-connecting, dreaming, and musing.

- **Rebirth, or spring/summer,** when your emotions will likely be more lively, boisterous, confident, and joyful. This is when your energy will likely be more outward, quick, clear, and fleet; and where your thoughts will likely be marked by daring, deciding, generosity, enjoyment, and moxie.

Then, put these stages of the death/rebirth cycle on your calendar, whether you use your computer, wall, or desk calendar. I personally like to color code fall/winter as purple and spring/summer as yellow. Using the stages of fall/winter and spring/summer that you have found for yourself, predict these stages out into the next six months. Tweak and adjust as you go through these months so you can really map out for yourself this death/rebirth cycle as it lives in you.

Ideally, you will be able to schedule more meetings, presentations, hot dates, vigorous exercise, and productivity spurts for your spring/summer stages. Add more acts of self-care, sleep, languid lovemaking, gentle forms of exercise, and extra time to dream for the fall/winter stages. And even if you have a packed, demanding schedule during a death phase, you will know that if you are barely keeping up, it is because you are momentarily out of alignment with your cycle, rather than not good enough, lazy, or crazy.

As I am writing this, my husband has texted me to remind me to send him possible dates for a two-day, grownups-only getaway, something we have been planning to do for a couple of months. He reminds me to pick a date as close to ovulation as possible and adds a smiley face emoticon. I scan the calendar on my computer, find the next yellow color-coded swath of days marked *spring/summer* and text him back a set of dates, also with a smiley face emoticon. That's tracking in action. Smiley face!

Look, I know that it can feel insane to go up and down and all around on rickety roller coasters in a world that's built for bullet trains. It can be crazy making to find yourself on the scenic route in a world that prefers getting swiftly from point A to point B. But aligning with your cycles helps to shift your perspective about the death part of the death/rebirth cycle. It helps you see that it is no mistake that you cycle, that cycling is, in fact, deliberate and intelligent. That you can't truly live without it. And that you will be a better woman for it.

And now, sister, it is time for more navigation skills, so you can not only become masterful at bearing your intense, "negative," or unwanted emotions, but so you can also find wisdom in the ugly, turn your devils into angels, and ask your shadow to show you the light.

When worked skillfully, traversing the dark will always reveal your light. But first, we must descend further.

death:
you can't live without it

7

Feel It, All of It
The Wisdom of Emotions—
And How to Not Die from Them

If you want to find happiness, you have
to make friends with unhappiness.
ANONYMOUS

hank you for all the ways you've been saying 'thank you' and
'please' and cooperating so well, love."

"You're welcome, Mama."

"It is so fun to be in a good mood together, right?"

"Yeah."

"But you know what? I love your grumpies and angries and sads,
too. I love being with you, no matter what mood you are in."

"Me, too, Mama. I like all the feelings."

I glance in the rearview mirror at my three-year-old cutie-pie. He
is looking content in his car seat, a ruby-lipped, curly-headed cherub
flown right off the ceiling of the Sistine Chapel, munching brown rice
crackers in my backseat.

You like all the feelings?

You. Like. *All*. The. Feelings?

I imagine his insides, his feelings. The whirlwind of excitement
when he shows me a new rocket ship tower he built out of magnetic
tiles. The gale of disappointment when I choose the wrong color bowl

to hold his snack of snap peas. The crashing waves of sadness when we can't find his stuffed animal, Lovie. Where did we leave Lovie? We can't go to sleep without Lovie!

I imagine that many of these times are the *first* time he has felt this particular emotion in his whole life. Loneliness. Longing. Rage. Grief. Indignation. Injustice. Bliss. Joy. Mischievousness. Contentment. Shame. Pride.

Amazingly, it seems as though he is learning to *like* and to *befriend* his feelings, which is pretty much opposite of what most of us learn early on, girls and boys alike. In fact, the arena of emotions—which ones are okay to have and which ones aren't, how much or how little is okay to express, or having emotions at all—is often a painful initiation in which we learn to constrict our self-expression, feel ashamed about what once felt natural, and secret away (into our shadow) the "unacceptable" parts of ourselves.

We learn things such as, what we feel doesn't matter. That our feelings disturb others, or are a form of manipulation. That if we have "bad" feelings, then we are "bad." That, ideally, we should never have any outbursts. That if we don't want to be left or punished, we'd better calm down—and how exactly do we do that? We shove our intense emotions into the wintery realms of our psyches, sidestep and avoid them wherever possible. We fix them, fade them, lighten them up, reason with them, attack them, or turn and run for our lives. It is a great understatement to say that we develop a limited repertoire in dealing with unwanted feelings in ourselves and in others.

In other words, we learn it is not safe to feel what we feel. One of my clients, Violette, tells me she was barely four years old when she realized that her father would never stop beating her with his leather belt and that, no matter what she felt about it, no one was coming to save her. She clearly remembers that moment as the first one when she sent her soul out of her body.

For Shelley, one of my mentees, there was no physical violence in her family, but she still internalized early on her family's concerns about what other people thought. She was eight years old when she traded her happy, playful self for a tough girl persona, learning that, in her family's code, you cover up your vulnerability with judgments and blame. In fact, she learned if you cover up what you are feeling with *doing*—staying busy, always achieving, and never slowing down—you don't have to feel at all. To-do lists and high earning became her favorite ways to numb herself.

So as we worked together, bit by bit, Shelley rewrote her inner critic as an inner cheerleader and rewrote her fear of vulnerability as emotional strength. Bit by bit, she eased up her self-punishment and extreme regimentation by re-introducing fun and silliness in her life. As she put it, "I got my childhood back."

Violette also shared with me that she doesn't know what to do with the immensity of her empathy and passion. She cares so deeply about the world that her circuitry shuts down until she can't feel much at all. How else can she make her way through a grocery store or dress her son for school without screaming like her hair is on fire, as she puts it? As is often the case for Violette, not knowing how to express the intense emotions of joy and ecstasy can be as bedeviling as not knowing how to deal with shame or rage. Given the choice between combusting from our intense emotions, or shutting down, most of us choose shutting down.

NAVIGATING EMOTIONAL STORMS

Regardless of our individual childhoods, almost all of us learn that our emotional storms are "tantrums"—irresponsible and immature outbursts that we would be able to manage if we weren't quite so deficient. We learn to numb to, and become ashamed of, the overwhelming physical sensations and restrictive beliefs that are associated with our emotions. I allow myself to wonder if it might turn out differently for my son—who likes all the feelings. I tear up when I hear him say this, because I myself am only beginning to really, truly, like all the feelings. I am proud that he might just be getting the hang of it some thirty years sooner than I've been able to.

As a new mom, however, I admit that I thought the best way to "manage" my son's toddler tantrums was to try to stop them, shorten them, or make them quieter. I told myself, "Just try not to lose your shit. Hold it all together. Or, just *look like* you are holding it all together." Also known as fix it, fade it, lighten it up, attack it, reason with it, or turn and run for your life.

But one afternoon when my two-year-old son exploded into a tantrum when a friend took a toy he was playing with, I tried something different. Instead of keeping my distance from his outburst, I pulled him close and held him, welcoming his feelings. I put on my inner galoshes and reminded myself that, although I might get very wet for the next bit of time, his emotional storm was not a problem.

I told him that I bet he was feeling sad and disappointed and probably angry, too. He looked at me thoughtfully. He pointed to his belly when I asked him where in his body he was feeling those things. When I asked him, "When she took your toy without asking, did it hurt your feelings?" he wailed *yes* and started crying some more. I didn't panic. I resisted the doubt that I had somehow made it worse or prolonged his agony. "Keep getting out the sads and the angries. Let the energy out," I instructed him.

I told him it made sense he was feeling sad, disappointed, angry, and hurt. I confirmed for him what happened: "Your feelings got hurt when she took away the toy you were playing with without asking." As he nodded, the storm started to downshift.

"You are feeling a lot, love. Feelings are strong. They are so much energy, aren't they?" Another vigorous nod. "How are you feeling now? Do you want me to dry your tears?"

"Not yet," he told me. "I want to cry some more."

And after a few more minutes, he asked me to dry his tears and told me he felt better now.

"Do you want to tell her that it hurt your feelings when she took your toy without asking and that you want her to ask you 'how many minutes' next time?" He nodded and went over to his little play pal and let out his truth. She said okay, she would next time. And offered him a turn with the toy.

What I practiced with my son is what I now practice with myself—and is what I wish I had learned when I myself was a girl child. And in a moment, I'll break down how you can practice it as well, with yourself or others, no matter how old. Tantrums can and must be redefined as intense emotional storms that, while they admittedly do overtake your body, soul, and mind in intense ways, hold important information for you. As Karla McLaren writes in *The Language of Emotions*, "Emotions are messages from our instinctive selves. . . . If we ignore and repress an emotion, we won't erase its message—we'll just shoot the messenger and interfere with an important natural process."[1] As you learn to surf your emotions and not drown in them—or at least when you *do* drown in them, to breathe underwater—you can then receive the truth that they are trying to deliver.

All faces of the feminine must be revered, without exception—even emotions. When I shared this at one of my retreats, I saw a light bulb turn on over Sian's head. Sian, a redhead whose presence is at once fiery and laid back, shared what that meant to her. "That means that my anger, my rage, my resentments, my fears, my hope, my passion, my beauty, and my ugly must all be revered—without exception." Over the course of the retreat, she was able to look at her emotions from this alternate perspective and to feel each part of herself, fully. This Feminine Genius skill teaches us how to feel "it," all of it, whatever *it* is, with ever more skill, wild abandon, and grace—and eventually with only intermittent bouts of self-destruction and a minor hemorrhage here and there.

I've come to understand that much of our suffering is optional. As I see it, most of our suffering, as women, as humans, stems from our inability to fully feel our feelings without attempting to escape them, numb them, drink them, shop them, eat them, caffeinate them, or smoke them away. When a storm gathers on the horizon, we have two very simple choices: number one, to put on our inner galoshes and feel it, all of it. Or number two, to self-destruct. More on transfiguring number two in the next chapter. More on number one now.

Feel All of It

> You get to keep all the strength
> and flexibility you are willing to feel.
> **DAVID SCHLUSSEL**

If you are anything like me or my clients, you also assume that if you fully feel your feelings, horrible, terrifying things will happen. You might actually die. You could be discovered as the fraud you suspect you are. You could be cast out of the family/tribe/group/sisterhood. You could turn to ash from shame. And you could be exposed as weak/not enough/ too much. So you think that the more you can resist *losing your shit* and the more you can *hold it all together*—or *look like you are holding it all together*—then you will stop having all these problematic *feelings*.

But. Until you can again feel what you feel, your life will never be your own.

Sian got more in-the-field practice with what she learned on retreat a few months later when her mother became mentally unstable and her father extremely physically ill. Sian dropped everything to be with them as her father died and it became necessary for her mother to go into a full-time care facility. For months, Sian ignored her feelings, got into adrenaline overdrive and stayed in it, focusing on all the things that needed to be done. But eventually, the tug of constant anxiety, blame, and nightmares got her attention. She realized it was time to feel her feelings, all of them.

Over minutes, days, and eventually months, she *leaned in* to her feelings rather than numbing them. She welcomed each emotion in turn, and began a dialogue with them, asking what wisdom they might have for her.

She began with the worst she could think of: blame. Sian felt vicious, her judgments of herself, and others, were rapier-sharp. This strange and ugly beast had her in its clutches and wouldn't let her go. Or, she couldn't let it go.

So Sian let herself wonder what could possibly be good about blame and the arrows it let her sling. She got curious about what its positive intention could possibly be for her. She nosed out the wisdom contained in blame's black heart, sure she would find some raw gem there.

She found it.

Blame, it turns out, is anger's scrappy sidekick. When anger's fire is too hot to hold, it will consume you, and blame understands this. More of an action than an emotion, blame's job is to direct some of anger's firepower out onto others, to buy you time until you can figure out what of that anger is for yourself, and what is truly for another. Blame's message for you is, *I'll stay with you until you can face the depth of your wounding and rage.*

Blame is a cry for help. A cry for help concealed in a battle cry, true, but a cry nonetheless. Sian's blame knew that if it could point out that it wasn't all her fault, that she was not alone in her family's perfect storm, then someone could be in it with her, notice her, notice her pain, come to her aid, and help.

Blame softened. Seen for its heroism rather than its villainy, it morphed. It shone a bit. It gave way to pure anger.

Sian inquired with curiosity into anger, and found that anger's message was, *something you value feels threatened.* "Oh. Something I *value,*" Sian pondered. "Something precious and dear to me is in danger, so anger hands me a sword to protect it." With this perspective, she felt into the white-hot heart of what she valued: Love, for her own sweet self. Love, for her family. Trust in life, and, if Sian was completely honest, mostly trust in herself.

Clear that Sian was now sharply aware of what she valued, anger happily tossed its mane and trotted off to become remorse. Remorse for losing her trust in herself and in life. Remorse put its arms around Sian, and they sank together into a pillow of sadness. *You lost something, something you cared about,* the sadness told her. Sian nodded. *That is what happened.* In sadness's embrace, she felt blameless in her blame. She felt tenderness for herself instead of anger. She felt pain, and she was exhausted, but she felt free.

As she did with blame and anger, Sian did with each of her dark emotions. She sniffed out each feeling's funky gifts, if only she would pause to unwrap them. She practiced how to not abandon herself (or self-destruct) at the onset of a storm, but instead, to *stay*.

Sian's anxiety, anger, self-doubt, and grief slowly but surely gave way to a sense of how loving, capable, okay, and rather wonderful she was. I see this time and time again: each emotion that is befriended, engaged with, bathed with curiosity, and then fully felt, likes to leave in its wake a side effect of self-esteem and wholeness.

The word *demon*, as in the monstrous doubts and compulsions we carry inside of us, comes from the word *daemon*, which means "the voice of your inner knowing." (Yeah, read that one again). Somewhere along the line, as pagan rites were tweaked by the Christian church, so were many important, sacred words. The word *daemon* that was known to mean a source of trustable inner guidance got twisted to mean instead the voices of evil inside you, utterly untrustable.

If you let them, your emotions will reveal themselves as daemons, not demons, as friends, not foes, and as guides, not saboteurs. They say, "This: try this. That: that is what is precious to you. There: go that way next." They will cup your face in their hands and turn you to see the pinhole of light—the proverbial light at the end of the tunnel. They will blow a little wind under your wings as you begin your ascent from the wintery underworld into the bright springtime.

Not quite convinced? As one of my mentors, Carla Camou, likes to remind me, the lifespan of an emotion is only between two to twenty minutes. Often, when you feel it fully and drink in the wisdom it contains, it passes of its own accord. Otherwise, when you deny it, wallow in it, or reacquire it, the emotion can stay dug in for a lifetime. The point of life isn't to stop having shit happen to you—*if* you want a life that feels right and true and well-lived and often quite fulfilling, that is. The ups and downs are not problems, nor are they indications you are doing it wrong. Problems will come. Strong, difficult, intense emotions will come. It is how you stay with them that is the key.

Imagine a woman who knows how to *feel it, all of it*, rather than shove her finger down her throat to stay thin, or have sex before she wants to in order to feel a facsimile of love. Imagine a woman who is in direct conversation with the sacred messages from All That Is.

She isn't having *tantrums*, she is feeling her feelings—also known as her truths, her values, her wants, her boundaries, her warning signals, and her fierce and tender loves.

Imagine a woman who knows that her feelings are the fiery, intense, wildly human reconfirmation of her divinity. Imagine a woman who no longer believes she is too much or not enough, but is just right. Imagine a woman who doesn't stop at, "I think, therefore I am" (thanks, Descartes), but continues on to, as my friend Annie Lalla likes to say, "I feel, therefore I am."

I have heard that our greatest fear as humans is a fear of death, but I don't completely agree. I think our greatest fear isn't just of dying, but also of being fully in life with all its ups and downs and unknowns and (seemingly) unbearables. We fear being too much, unloved, outcast, not enough, sick, insane, a burden, heartbroken, and abandoned, and we think that the problem with these fears is that we could die from—or keep having to live with—the physical and emotional pain of them.

What do we humans know of actual death? We can only know death when we die, and then it is (probably) too late to report back. We only know life; and in life, we fear change, intensity, chaos, uncertainty, loss, shock, surprise, shame, and even our huge swells of rapture and power. We even fear garden-variety contentment, especially if it lasts too long and makes us forget our to-do lists. We fear what we feel.

One of our greatest tasks then becomes to gaze at each bedeviling feeling right in its bedeviling little eye and say, "Take me. I'm yours."

Emotions aren't a bug in the programming, something left over from your malfunctioning lizard brain or incomplete childhood. You do not have these weird, unwieldy emotions that happen mysteriously to you, and you simply need to tolerate them, like that crazy uncle you have to sit next to at Thanksgiving dinner. Your emotions aren't a mistake; they are some of the best parts of you. Feelings aren't a design flaw; they are divine in origin. You are not a weakling because you have intense emotions; your ability to feel them fortifies your inner knowing and strengthens your physical body as you walk the often-intense path of Feminine Genius.

And here is how you welcome in each wily comrade and practice feeling it—all of it.

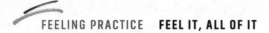

FEELING PRACTICE   FEEL IT, ALL OF IT

1 Welcome each emotion.
2 Let it pierce you to your bones.
3 Wait.
4 Mine for the gem of wisdom in each emotion.

Let me say more about each step.

Welcome each emotion. By *welcome*, I mean that you take on the stance of inviting rather than resisting your emotions—as though you were saying, "Come in, you are welcome here."

Welcoming each emotion is an attitude, a stance. If ordinarily you tense up and feel dread at the onset of an emotion, see if you can instead open your mind and heart and body to it. When you find yourself reaching to drink, shop, purge, eat, cut, smoke, drug, whatever—pull back your urge and stay put. Invite each emotion to sit with you in your inner salon as a welcome guest.

Strong, intense, and "negative" emotions are part of life. Stuff that you don't want to happen, happens. To everyone. It always will. And while this might indicate something is "wrong" or misaligned in your life, it never indicates that something is wrong with *you*.

Let it pierce you to your bones. I first heard the phrase "Let it pierce you to your heart" from the Buddhist nun Pema Chödrön, who was speaking about navigating scary, hard stuff. Let the emotion—and all the bodily sensations that it rides in on—pierce you to the very epicenter of your breastbone. Instead of damming up your feelings or collapsing your chest, take down the levee and let the emotion flood through your body and bones, absolutely and completely. Let it do its thing.

Breathing is good. Crying is good. Shaking is great. Swearing, sweating, pacing, yelling, panting, dancing, lying face down on the cold floor—all superb.

Get the grumpies and the angries and the sads out. Let them have their way with you and let them be through with you when they are through with you. Grumpies and angries and sads like completing their natural cycle, and they will mess with you big time if you rush them. The more you relax, the more you *lean in* and *open* to the feeling rather than contracting, panicking, or running the other way, the more you let it get all the way into each nerve fiber of your body, the sooner it will release you. Counterintuitive, but true. Remember, the lifespan of any emotion is anywhere between two to twenty minutes. Just that.

This bone-piercing step is here to remind you to simply stop yourself from automatically running away from unwanted emotions, however intense it is to let them course through your body and being. As you let the arrows of your feelings burst your breastbone, I suggest you ask yourself and your body questions like, "What am I feeling? What sensations? Where in my body am I feeling them? Tell me more. What is this like for me? What's important about it? Tell me more."

Instead of using your mind and thoughts to talk yourself *out* of whatever you are feeling and *into* a cigarette, a joint, a latte, a shopping trip, or binge-watching Netflix, use your mind to catalogue the sensations and locations of the feelings. Rather than using your mind to *escape* as quickly as possible, use your mind and thoughts to *be there* along with your feelings. Do something revolutionary: partner up these often-warring parts of yourself—your body, your feelings, and your mind.

Resist the urge to panic if your emotion swells instead of ebbs. Resist the urge to believe you have made it worse by *leaning in*. Often, when you are "freaking out" or "triggered" or "looping endlessly" on a big emotion, you have "age regressed." Meaning, it is as though you have gone back in time to when you were three or four years old, or younger. You are literally re-experiencing your feelings from when you were about my son's age, or Violette's age when she sent her soul away, or Shelley's age when she traded her happy girl self for her tough girl self.

This whole step allows you to take yourself into your own arms, cradle yourself, and go absolutely nowhere. It offers you peace with yourself and with life, and has nothing to do with transcending or sanitizing anything. I mean, in the next moment of your life, there is just as likely to be a joy storm as a shit storm. This kind of peace has everything to do with the kind of radiant self-acceptance that is emergent when we don't run from whatever it is that we feel.

Wait. A deep inhalation. The calm of the storm pausing or stopping: wait for this.

Wait means you need to stay put until the moment your system shifts from I'm-freaking-out mode to I-am-okay mode. Perhaps there will be a physical sign like the impulse to take a deep breath (as my son did after his storm downshifted), or an intuitive sense that something has completed. It is important to remember that emotions have a natural life cycle. If you wait, your emotions can surge, ebb, and then naturally complete. This is the most respectful way I know of to *calm down*.

So, wait for it.

Mine for the gem of wisdom in each emotion. This step might come in the short lull directly after the storm of feelings, or later in the day or week. I suggest you mine for the gem of wisdom in the emotion by asking, "What are you trying to tell me?" Pretty straightforward.

Even if you have felt deep shame for your feelings, you can develop an outright reverence for all emotions. I think of them

Core Messages of Emotions

Fear	There is potential danger here.
Anger	There is a (real or imagined) threat to something you value.
Sadness	Something you value is lost.
Grief/Heartbreak	Something you had your whole heart in is gone.
Despair	You think you can't do it.
Envy/Jealousy	You see something you want for yourself.
Annoyance/Disgust	It isn't the way you want it to be.
Loneliness	You need or want connection (with others or yourself).
Depression	The way you have set up your life isn't working.
Confidence	You can do it.
Joy	This is something you love and fills you with life-force.
Happiness	You like what you are experiencing right now.
Gratitude	You are receiving something greater than yourself.
Panic	You think it is going to get worse, and you are not going to be able to handle it.
Anxiety	It could go wrong, or it could be okay.
Guilt	Something you have done could have (or has) displeased another.
Shame	You feel that something about you or something you did is wrong. Something is out of alignment.

as message-bringers from your soul's headquarters. Each one is a bearer of a truth—a gift—that you are apparently now ready to unwrap. But you have to unwrap it. Emotions are gems of wisdom encased in wild and wooly packaging. It takes something to stay lucid long enough to get under their tough skin to their rich interiors. In order not to spontaneously combust from the heat of your emotions, you must develop the unwavering belief that each is wise, not flawed.

So, ask each emotion what its message is, ask each feeling what its wisdom is. And then listen. Try, "Hello, emotion. What is the wisdom you are bringing? What is the core message you are trying to convey to me?"

Use the Core Messages of Emotions table on the previous page, inspired by my mentor Carla Camou, as a guide to help you mine the wisdom waiting for you at the epicenter of your emotions. This list is guidance, not gospel. It is not complete, but has some of the biggies. It might be spot on for you, or way off base. Ultimately, go with what you hear within yourself.

Asking each emotion what its message is will also help you get clear on *what happened*. Simply naming what happened can help the storm subside, as it did for my son. It can help a part of you feel heard, seen, acknowledged, and understood, as it did for Sian. Take note that this step is not about *why* what happened, happened. Asking *why* is generally counterproductive, often whips up new emotional storms, and usually diverts your attention from the wisdom within your original emotion. Stay with: *Yes, that is what happened. Yes, what happened was witnessed.*

Once you begin to unwrap the anger, the grief, the fear, or the envy, you can begin to see what is so valuable to you that you would protect it ruthlessly from threat (anger's message), what it is that you have loved and lost (grief), where you are smelling potential danger (fear), and what that something *is* that you dearly want for yourself (envy).

This process of self-inquiry must come first. After you open the gift of the emotion, eventually, it will become clear what you want to express about these feelings you felt, these discoveries you made, these truths that revealed themselves to you. Self-inquiry fist, expression second. (And expression practices are coming up in part four.)

Each emotion comes to show you your next step on the path. Inspired by my friend Annie "I-feel-therefore-I-am" Lalla, I see your feelings as angelic messengers sent from the other world into your world, telegrams from your future self to your current self. But because feelings come before language and before reason, and because they communicate through sensation, you must practice decoding each emotion with curiosity, kindness, and tenacity.

Then feelings as tough as rage, blame, depression, and grief can open their shells and reveal the pearls inside.

feel it, all of it,
or you will miss your life

8

Going Down

Mining for Gold in a Dark Night of the Soul

Soul work is not a high road. It is a deep fall into
an unforgiving darkness that won't let you go
until you find the song that sings you home.
McCALL ERICKSON

On a chilly November morning, I got a Facebook message from a woman named Sarah, thanking me for a recent interview. What struck her was not that I had focused on the light, bright, high-flying parts of our femininity, even though they are vital. She thanked me for my courage in talking frankly about the down-and-dirty, dark descent parts of the death/rebirth cycle.

It's true. To see that failed plans can also be part of the grand plan requires you to *climb down* from your high horse. Aligning with your cycles, to claim not only your rebirths but also your deaths, requires you at some point to *descend*. Opening the basement door to your shadowy emotions, digging up disowned parts of yourself, and welcoming each as a long-buried and long-lost friend, requires you to *go deep*. Likewise, finding gold in something so raw and brutal as a dark night of the soul is at first an unexpected, disorienting drop into unimaginable depths.

down, girl, down

GOING DOWN

It was 6:00 a.m. I blinked, then opened my eyes begrudgingly. *You are going down today,* my inner voice informed me.

No, I decide. I'll be okay today. I'll just ignore my pesky inner voice and focus on the light. In fact, maybe it wasn't my inner voice at all, but the voice of doubt, or fear. *Yeah, that's what it is,* I reasoned, *just illusory fear and doubt.*

A natural hermit, I was then living in a house in a busy urban area with two toddlers and five adults who all worked from home. I was breast-feeding, a new mom, and I'd begun my sleep-deprivation marathon with an emergency C-section. My decade-long, rock-solid marriage was shaky. I also had recently returned to work. I was physically and metaphysically depleted; and the foods, supplements, and practices that had, throughout my life, kept me healthy and thriving no longer helped. I would try to breathe, meditate, focus on pleasure, and summon gratitude for my amazing life. But my time-tested tools for shifting my experience failed me. My tank was empty, and I was choking on that particular kind of sediment that is only found at the very bottom of an empty tank. And I didn't know how to fill up.

My inner voice wasn't messing around. Again, it portended emphatically: *Listen. Today is* not *going to be a good day!*

I just didn't want to hear it. *Not one of these days again,* I prayed. Please.

For a year, *one of these days* had descended upon me like a dark swarm, moving swiftly across the horizon, leaving no leaf or twig standing in its wake. *One of these days* could often become ten, a wild pack of days that hunted me and took me down at the knees.

For a year, I had spent *one of these days* after *one of these days,* kneeling, wondering what poison I'd unwittingly drunk. Kneeling, as you do at a pew, an altar, a shrine, a toilet. "Please, God," I prayed, "What is wrong with me? Where did I go? What did I do wrong to feel this, and what can I do right to stop feeling this? Please, God, make it stop. God, are you there? God?"

I wondered if I was having panic attacks. I would shake so fiercely that I had to put down the car keys. I would put on a sweater in mid-summer to help with the chill in my bones.

I wondered if I was going through early menopause. I would wake in the dead of night from dreams of dying, the sheets soaked. I would stroll through an ordinary moment, then suddenly double over, sobbing.

I wondered if this was what it felt like to slowly lose your mind. Everything looked flat and lifeless. I felt nothing in my body when my husband touched me. I could remember, almost, that I was beautiful and capable. But then my conviction would slide, evaporate.

I wondered if I'd always had this ominous white noise on the inside, if I'd always felt so toxic and ugly, but just never noticed. Forget about getting through the day, how would I get through this next minute? Was it cancer? Chronic fatigue? A brain tumor? Was I crazy? Had my Feminine Genius forsaken me?

Yes. For a year, *one of these days* descended on me. Again. And again. And again. And no amount of kneeling or praying or focusing on the light would help.

In the physical, material world, I consulted doctors and healers who found that I was experiencing depression, low thyroid functioning, adrenal fatigue, an autoimmune disorder of my insulin, chronic inflammation, and toxic levels of lead and mercury.

In the metaphysical, soul world, my self-esteem had fallen and could not get up. My emotions raged and abated without me understanding why they started or when they would stop. The war inside myself had returned. I was inspired to do my work in the world, but my body wasn't strong enough to hold my calling. My cauldron was cold, lacking fire to transfigure these dark ingredients.

I didn't know what to do, and no one else did either. My husband and the friends I lived with tried to help, mostly by trying to fix it, fade it, lighten it up, attack it, reason with it, or turn and run for their lives—what anyone does who is uneducated in the ways of the dark. As

I was fixed, faded, lightened, attacked, reasoned with, and run from, I became a self-fulfilling prophecy. The more lonely I felt, the more I isolated myself. The more the war raged inside me, the more my husband and I fought. The more I doubted myself, the more my community became doubtful of how to help.

Utterly exhausted, my personal churches caught fire and burned. My connection with my husband that I had polished daily like a golden idol crumbled. My trust in my friends, community, and sisters to help when I needed it most went up in flames. My confidence in my intuition, my body, and my ability to speak the truth even when hard blackened and charred. I looked over the landscape of my heart and saw only ashes where cathedrals had once blazed with holy light.

The things I had called sacred went missing, trailing off into the twilight.

One friend asked me if she should worry about me hurting myself. I thought about how I wished to not be here, to stop being constantly reminded what a waste of space I was. I thought about how I longed for my days to be other than full of wracked pain. I wondered if I would ever feel good again. But the truth was I was too tired to research options for offing myself. I learned that there are different kinds of suicidal ideations and mine was the kind where I wanted to just make it stop. Not to do myself harm, but to just: Make. The Burning. Stop.

Apprentice to the Queen of the Dark

Unwittingly, I had become an apprentice to the Queen of the Dark—my affectionate name for the dark aspect of Feminine Genius, a weather witch of the highest order. The part of the path she pushed me onto was unpaved, unlit, and uncharted, littered with the wounded parts of myself I could have sworn I had already healed. Although I know now that it is part of the path that most of us are pushed onto at some point in our lives, at the time I felt alone, broken, and crazy.

When it comes to walking the path of Feminine Genius, what you knew yesterday is not what you need to know today. The Queen of the Dark levels everything, so you can know again and afresh.

"Excuse me, Queen? Um, how am I supposed to stay standing while everything is collapsing? How am I supposed to trade up *who I was* for *who I am becoming*? And um, Queen, how am I supposed to turn lead into gold when I've got no fire for my cauldron?"

She said nothing, just held my gaze and handed me a stick so I could stir the ashes.

The winter the Queen had pushed me into was different from any other winter I had previously made it through. Not only its duration and intensity—months stacked upon months—but its flavor. It tasted to me of spiritual wasteland. My familiar landmarks had disappeared. What had previously worked well was now of no use. I felt deeply alone, and not just separate from my fellow human beings, but separate from All That Is. I had fallen far into a *bardo*—a state of suspended animation after death yet before one's next birth—where even the ever-present light of the Divine could not find me. This, I came to understand, is known as a *dark night of the soul*.

It turns out that a rebellious Spanish monk named Saint John of the Cross coined the phrase "dark night of the soul." As Mirabai Starr, who writes about Saint John of the Cross and other Christian mystics, describes it:

> In a dark night of the soul . . . all the ways you have become accustomed to tasting the sacred dry up and fall away. All concepts of the Holy One evaporate. You are plunged into a darkness so impenetrable that you are convinced it will never lift. You may flail about for something—anything—to prop you up, but you grasp only emptiness. And so, rendered reckless by despair, you let yourself fall backward into the arms of nothing.
>
> This, according to John of the Cross, is a blessing of the highest order.[1]

During my year of hell, well-meaning friends would say, "What doesn't kill you makes you stronger." "Everything happens for a reason." "This too shall pass." "You're going to laugh at this and have one hell of a story to tell." "It is always darkest before the dawn." "Keep your chin up. Just smile. You are strong." I knew they meant well and were probably right, but I spat out their benedictions in disgust.

I fell back into the arms of nothing. A blessing of the highest order? This was like no grace I knew, thanks anyway.

What brings on a dark night of the soul, how long it lasts, and what a dark night feels like while you are in one varies from woman to woman, but it has a special seat in the salon of the underworld. A dark night of the soul can often show its face as depression, dissociation (feeling "out of your body"), anxiety, chronic physical and emotional pain, sudden change, the death of someone you loved, a betrayal, or a loss like that of your relationship, job, community, income, or home. What distinguishes a dark night of the soul from a garden-variety dark time is that it is about, well, your soul.

On the path to wholeness, your soul (also known as Feminine Genius) won't stand for any bypassing and will instead route you deliberately through your shit. You can get ahead in life by ignoring and mistreating your body, but to be on the path of Feminine Genius requires you to embrace and venerate your body. What at first may blacken your interior landscape will eventually build new castles. What at first feels like an affliction or abandonment by your soul will eventually come to feel like fortification and a renewal of your soul.

Which is all admittedly damn near impossible to keep in mind while you are *in* a dark night of the soul.

If You Are in a Dark Night of the Soul *Right Now*

So if you, my friend, are mid-spiral right now, on your way down, or all the way down, know that the dark place you are in, where it seems God herself has forsaken you—I have been there. I may be there again. And I am listening. Even if I never get to meet you, I will meet you here.

Because the dark is a place where I made my home and found my Home, I can go there with you now, anytime. I can sit with you, and you will feel the metronome of my heart beating with yours. We can burn, together. I know how to burn with you, yet not go down in flames. I am educated in the ways of the dark. I made it out alive, and you will, too. And not just alive, but *alive. Re-birthed.* The parts of you dying in there, you don't need them anymore, not where you are going.

If you are there right now, I know you can barely hear me. I know sound is muffled, and anything that tastes remotely of a platitude, you will spit out at once. But hear this: Where you are, is not a mistake. You are in the forge. The Goddess of Holy Blacksmithery knows what the hell she is doing. I myself have no map or script or blueprint to give you, but you will still make your way through.

But don't worry about that now. It might sound like bullshit. Just put one foot in front of the other. Breathe in and breathe out. Again. And again. Don't even try to imagine the sacred yet. I will not try to convince you there is any sacred left in your life. Just give me your hand and take one more step with me, and then one more. I know that where we are going is worth all of it, but you don't have to believe me. All you have to do is trust me. You don't even have to trust me—just stay with me.

Stay with me here. I know you want to go. I know you want it to end, and I know that things that would ordinarily horrify you are starting to sound good right about now, if they would just: Make. The. Burning. Stop. I know you wonder if you are crazy, if this is what it feels like when a mind turns itself inside out, shakes itself of its contents, and returns to the wild.

Stay with me here. Let me show you what can help. Let me show you where the cracks are in the fortress without cracks. Let me show you the rungs on the ladder out of the cesspool you are submerged in. Let me straighten the crown on your head as you dodge arrows flying at you from your own mouth.

Stay with me here. Keep reading. Keep feeling. There will be at least one good, true, and useful thing you will find here that will work for you. Let me show you how to use pain as a life raft. Let me show you the wisdom of what feels insanely hard. Let me show you how to let your isolation drag you into the arms of the Beloved.

Apprenticing to the Queen of the Dark brings fresh humility to your heart. She will renew your confidence in your body, your desires, and your inner voice. Hanging out with shadows, where the maps have all been torn up and the signposts have all been torn down, letting the wisdom contained within every terrible thing show itself to you, allows you to chart a way through. You and I have more to do in the coming chapters, but now it is time to pull out your cauldron and your stirring stick.

In a dark night of the soul, you look out over your scorched earth, recognizing nothing, hearing only the loud absence of all you have held close. Let me show you how this is indeed a blessing of the highest order. Let me show you what the fuck to do when you go down into the dark night in the death/rebirth cycle.

Stay with me here. Let me show you how to grab another and another and another pearl out of the underworld and return to this world, *alive*. You are in a holy place, even though it feels like hell. This is where an aspect of your Genius is birthed.

WAKING UP IN THE DARK

> Change the way you look at things
> and the things you look at change.
> **WAYNE DYER**

On one of my all-time worst days, I somehow drove across a bridge and through a maze of freeways to meet with a friend, a gifted poet and artist, Kate. Her mane of blond curls backlit by the sunset, she greeted me on the street outside the French bistro where she suggested we meet.

She took one look in my eyes and said, "Oh, sweetie. You don't look good. You are really going through it, aren't you?" She had simply named what was happening. I relaxed a tiny bit.

She walked alongside me as we made our way to the restaurant, listening. I could feel her heart near to mine, also listening. Occasionally, she would speak and ask me more about what I was feeling, what it meant to me, what had happened, who else knew? The clouds lifted a tiny bit. Over steak frites and a shared glass of burgundy, a deep red elixir shot with bright stars, she listened. A quiet, yet alive kind of listening. She stayed with me in my ravaged condition. She offered her curiosity about what I was going through. And sometimes she shared about when she had gone through similar times. She handed me tissues, but not advice.

Kate has a rare gift: the capacity to be with someone who is in the dark, and to listen. To meet them there, naked and innocent. To feel what they are feeling along with them, then burn with them in the full agony of it, but somehow not lose herself in the burning. To inquire gently into their experience, to ask questions powered only by curiosity, not judgment. To be so at ease with her own emotional range that she is okay to be with someone else who is at the bottom register of their own. Never did she try to fix it, fade it, lighten it up, attack it, reason with it, or turn and run for her life.

Kate, educated in the ways of the dark, silently assumed there was rightness and intelligence in my experience. She knew that this kind of intelligence never presents reasons first. It shows up as feelings, sensations, and intuition that can be ciphered into reasons only after they have been dosed with respect. She looked at my darkness yet still saw beauty. My demons and I stopped feeling so wretched. Kate was a balm. I received her grace. My shame and I took one long last pained exhale and slowly sat back in the chair, at rest.

That evening, a touch tipsy, a Feminine Genius named Kate spilled some dawn all over my dark night. She reminded me of everything I already knew but had forgotten. That just because something was wrong in my life, didn't mean that *I* was wrong. That even though there were certainly things out of alignment inside me and in my life, I was still whole. That there was nothing about me to be ashamed of, and that even my shame was beautiful. She allowed me to see myself the way she saw me: precious, a wonder; utterly and joyously loved.

Ignited by the grace of my friend, a part of my self woke up.

A few months later, on a cold, brilliant New Year's Eve night, my inner voice again spoke up clearly: *This journey through the underworld is complete. You're coming up.*

GOING DOWN AND COMING UP

As I see it, dark nights of the soul are a kind of soul software update. Your soul needs to remind you from time to time to see yourself as Feminine Genius sees you: precious, a wonder; utterly and joyously loved. The re-birth that can come after a dark night of the soul is designed to bring you more wholly alive, even if it does so by nearly killing you.

As a culture, we have huge resistance to going down. We avoid it, caffeinate it, and medicate it. Because down is where our shadow is, our shame is, our pain and wrath and greed and gluttony. Down is where we tossed our true selves when we learned they weren't welcome, perhaps as far back as act 1. Down is where up is down and down is further down and we lose our eyesight and have to feel our way through. Down is where our creeping, crawling demons lie, where our disowned and ugly parts live still. Down is broken hearts and festering wounds. Down is death, down is dark, down is no life.

And yet.

Remember Riya from a few chapters back? Drunk on a rainy Friday night, holding a DUI ticket in her shaking hands? Feeling like she was dying inside, trying to numb with alcohol and food the pain she felt each day at work and with her family? That night and the year after were the hardest she had ever been through.

Riya found me six years later, well into her work with healers and therapists, and on her way out of her dark night. She had spent a lifetime stomping out not only her intuition but also her real and natural desires that deserved to be honored. She examined her restrictive beliefs and was able to see that "I'm bad, I'm crazy, and I'm wrong" were false beliefs, never true. She realized she was able to become someone she never thought she could be: herself.

With her dark night of the soul in her rearview mirror, Riya could see that without her descent, she would still be in a soul-sucking corporate job, ignoring the problems in her marriage, and trying to be who she felt she was supposed to be while rebelling against it all. She wrote to me recently, "My dark night gave me the kick in the pants and the courage I needed to step into who I came here to be. I had to change. If I didn't change, I would have destroyed myself and maybe others, and that is not okay with me. I needed to evolve myself as though my life depended on it, because it did and does."

One wish that Feminine Genius—the collective soul—has for you is to heal any split you have within yourself. As Riya found, the more you gaze into your shadow, the less potential you have to unwittingly hurt others. Since a cage doesn't always look like a cage at first, a dark night of the soul can pry open your eyes to whatever cage you find yourself in. It can act like a detox program, removing the crutches of addictive behaviors and strengthening your own legs to work again.

Some blessings only feel like blessings way after the fact. Sian describes her dark night of the soul as having demons pour hot tea on her, turn into angels, and then put ice packs on the sore spots. After the death of her father, she found herself in her own midlife, childless in a close circle of friends with lots of babies, without her own clear direction, and feeling lost inside. She felt she had been here before, was lost again, but this time couldn't shake it. On the outside things looked amazing—a loving husband, a beautiful home in a beautiful city, all her needs met. But for two years she could barely tolerate being alive.

Sian shared with me, "I do not embrace the dark times while they are happening. There is a cloak, a shield, that comes over me and I can't see clearly." And yet, the perspective of embracing rather than rejecting not only her demons, but also all parts of herself, gradually brought her some power and peace. Her rebirth has been her consciously choosing to stay alive and do more cool things with her life. Her main understanding is that even though there is so much darkness on this material plane, she doesn't actually have to be afraid of it. The dark night may come multiple times. It is dirty, messy, and it hurts. And we are okay after. We are better for it. We are not alone.

She says sagely, "I definitely am not taking things as seriously anymore, and I see most of our human experience as an illusion, a game, a play of Leela for our souls to learn what they need to and keep moving on and evolving into more light. I am so grateful to know this. And"—she smiles wryly—"it is a lot easier to see this when we are out of the dark time and back in the light."

There is nothing spiritually superior about experiencing a dark night of the soul over a straightforward heartache or a really bad mood. They all belong in the emotional season of winter. All are a stripping away, a going within, a desperate swimming through cold waters. It often takes a great time of darkness to spawn a great beginning. All bulbs take root in the fertile void of wintertime. But a dark night of the soul stands apart because of the feelings of abandonment by life itself that you suffer—and then reconcile.

Battered, breathless, wild-eyed because we have seen some shit, we—Riya, Sian, and I—are able to write home about it because we have been mercifully tossed back on the shore of the living. For now.

Mining for Gold in the Dark

The dark is the fertile void, the Earth herself, a womb, a cauldron, where creativity gets its start. After a heroic lap or two on your Heroine's Journey, you reach a hand—or your whole body—into the fertile void, and the hand of the Divine reaches back. *Oh, the descent, it's a tricky business,* the Divine Darkness says. *Here's a pearl, and here's another. Now, go, string these together and offer them to the world.*

What is a blessing of the highest order? What or who is at cause for the moments of grace that propel our darkest times into their eventual completion?

Maybe for Sian it was a woman she didn't even know in West Africa or Pakistan or Paris who had pulled herself up by her own bootstraps out of her own dark time and placed a self-made crown on her own head, and these actions undulated throughout space and time, piercing Sian's frozen heart.

Maybe for Riya it was her own future self, who had already and completely integrated the understanding of her dark time, and who had traveled back in an altruistic quantum leap to play the role of personal guardian angel, whispering truth so that Riya could build herself a new North Star.

Maybe for me it was my husband and close friends. Not the obvious day-to-day parts of them that were in just as much pain as

I was, but the metaphysical parts of them that came into this life and created our relationship "contract," not just to stand for fun times but also to stand fiercely for my freedom, my self-love, my sovereignty. In fact, their stand for me was so fierce that they were willing to construct a gauntlet that would nearly kill me, but didn't. It was one that required of me to become the woman I was aching to become.

Maybe for you it will be a stanza of a poem or a line from a book that lodges like an ember in your heart at the appropriate time in your misery, and fireworks its medicine throughout your dimmed insides, warming you again.

My prayer is for all of us to audaciously assume that miracles are always aimed in our direction, to recognize them where we used to walk right by them, and to remember that grace comes in many forms, including homemade soup on your doorstep, a smile from a stranger, kind listening, a scalpel, a dark night of the soul. As Nisargadatta Maharaj, an Indian teacher of non-dualism says, "The other world is this world, rightly seen." It is good to remember that we need as much schooling in navigating the dark as in cultivating the light, to help us wipe away the film over our eyes so we can rightly see.

The Queen of the Dark knows that often, as writer Mirabai Starr notes, "pain is the cure for pain."[2] A dark night of the soul removes all facsimiles of power so you can taste the real deal for yourself. Going down fortifies your body and psyche so that you don't scare easily from your truth, and helps you build stamina for another lap on the path of Feminine Genius. The descent drops you off, naked, in a dark forest in the middle of the journey of your life, and helps you find your way home.

> Whatever the name of the catastrophe,
> it is never the opposite of love.
> **MARY OLIVER, "SHADOWS"**

GOING DOWN PRACTICE MINING FOR GOLD IN A DARK NIGHT OF THE SOUL

Note: If you are in the middle of a dark night of the soul now, you might want to skip this practice and come back to it later. Really. Don't get me wrong. It is a great practice. But if, as you look it over, you notice your middle finger raising in my direction, you are likely too deeply *in* a current dark time to have any useful perspective *on* your current dark time. So either pick an event further back in your past, head back to chapter 7 to the "Feel It, All of It" exercise, or skip to the next chapter, "Navigating Storms: A Cheat Sheet," for bite-sized help, instead.

Otherwise, take a moment to sit quietly and put a hand on your body. I always favor my low belly not only because it brings my awareness out of my head and into my body, but also because many consider the belly to be the place in the body where the soul is most concentrated. It is here, to your very core, that you ideally will *direct* the following questions; and it is from here that you'll ideally feel you *receive* answers. Notice your breath as it travels *inside* your body, almost as though it is giving your insides a gentle caress.

Ask yourself the following questions, one by one, and then write or record the answers you hear:

1 Describe a dark night of the soul in your past. If you can't locate one, a great disappointment, heartbreak, or personal rock bottom will do just fine.

2 When it was at its most painful, in what ways were you most challenged?

3 Looking back, what can you see now that you couldn't see then?

4 What aspect of your strength and your authority has only become available because of going through it?

5 In what ways is it a blessing?

Only to the extent that we expose ourselves
over and over to annihilation, can that
which is indestructible in us be found.
PEMA CHÖDRÖN, *When Things Fall Apart*

Sister, when you find yourself in that dark place, where there is only shadow, and the walls are too tall to let in light, know that I have been there.

Yes, it can feel like you are dying, because you *are* dying.

Yes, it can feel like you can't do it, because you *can't*.

The part of you that got you here to the door of the dark is not the part of you that will jailbreak you out. That part of you that brought you here will be burned alive. Ashes. That part is surely dying, and a new part, beaten and shaped by the black flames of the bellows, is emerging.

And she—she is resplendent. Refined, sovereign, two feet planted authoritatively on the Earth. She has seen some shit.

And her diamond eyes are clear and flashing.

I would not trade this burning for all the
wine in the world, for it has transfigured me,
and now I am made of holy fire.
MIRABAI STARR, *Saint Teresa of Avila: Passionate Mystic*

9

Navigating Storms
A Cheat Sheet

Barn's burnt down.
Now I can see the moon.
MIZUTA MASAHIDE

I f the previous chapter was a lot to swallow, here are some bite-sized nuggets to remind you how far you have come and to help you go even further.

What Kills You Makes You Stronger   Down, death, dark, descent; they are your friends, even if at first it seems they will kill you. They will, in fact, kill a part of you. Whatever part you no longer need, let it burn away. Don't stop at the surface. Go deep. Plant your seeds in the most fertile soil, so that a new—and stronger—part can be born.

What Goes Down, Must Come Up   Your ups and downs are not curses. Your cycles, calling to you from the province of nature, connect you to your natural wisdom. Like the moon and the stars, yours is a heavenly body. As any heroine can see, you may not need to be medicated; you might just need to align yourself with your cycles.

Don't Bypass Anything; Just Put One Foot in Front of the Other   When you are through your dark time, you will look back and be able to see it for the lesson, the growth, the great story, the silver lining, and even the blessing that it is. While you are in it, you will not.

For now, just swim one more stroke, just hoe one more row, just take one more breath. Feel it, all of it. Keep it moving. Let the river of your feelings rage over your internal sandbags or dams. Or trickle, or evaporate like fog on a hot day. However it moves, let it. Let it have you.

It has to go somewhere. When you stop its flood, it burrows deep in your mind, in your heart, in your tissues, bones, and blood. And it rots. That kind of decay can make you unwell. Don't let it fester. Compost that shit and let it flow.

Tend to Your Girl Child   Every emotional storm you experience wallops both a past version of you along with a present-day version of you. The current storm reminds you of a past storm. Or, the current storm invokes the beliefs you made in a past storm, or the current storm makes you feel as small and vulnerable as you did when you really *were* small and vulnerable—and probably couldn't even wipe your own butt yet.

So, imagine a freaked-out younger version of you that is also having this stormy experience with you. Scoop her into your arms, like I did with my son on the playroom floor.

Tell this little, frightened part of you, "I've got you. You're okay." Feel what it feels like to hold your girl-child self in your arms and in your lap. Feel the little one's storm begin to downshift.

Then, imagine you are the little one. Feel what it is like to *be held* by strong arms and to be in a safe lap. Imagine yourself reclining into a body that is strong and loving. If that's a bit of a somatic tongue twister, it is meant to be. Don't worry, you've got this. You can be both adult woman and girl child at once.

Take Your Breaks   When you catch a break, or when you need to create one so you can pull yourself together just to take out the trash, go grocery shopping, care for your kids, or work on your novel, I suggest this: *bracket it. Bracketing* is a term that comes from psychology that means to put your emotional storm inside brackets [like these].

With bracketing, you don't *bury* your emotions, you don't pretend they are not there, you don't ignore or wish them away. Instead you put them on a shelf for later. You promise them (and yourself) that you will be back with your full attention, but for now, you need to focus on something else. And then later, make good on that promise, and un-bracket your dark.

If You Can, Enlist Help Ask a friend, or even pay someone if that is available to you, to feed you, remind you to shower, make a list of the supplements you need to take and when, come with you to doctors' appointments, water the plants, take the kids to the park, hold your hand, help you make sense of it all, or see past your shame to your beauty.

It is hard to be the only one tracking your well-being when you are in the dark, because being in the dark tends to spiral you further into the dark. But you have to reach out. Ask. It is a sign of strength, not of weakness. Your friends and family will respect and trust you more for asking, not less. Regardless of what they have on their plates, your request will require them to tap into a resourceful, sturdy, and compassionate place within them—a place that they might not be able to access except through your asking.

Reach out and ask. But give them guidelines such as, "Don't ask how I am; just silence." "Let's watch a movie." "No advice, please; just listen." "Bring take-out Thai food." "Massage my feet." "Don't say, 'Let me know what I can do.' I don't know what I need, so ask me questions and we'll find it together." "Hug me and let me be the one to pull away first." "Remind me it is going to be okay."

Treating each other with dignity while we navigate the dark, and even treating dark times as a healthy part of being alive, is a rare and nascent skill set for most humans. Most people want to help, but don't know how. Throw them whatever bone you can.

String Your Pearls As you complete your alchemical journey through the underworld, you will have composted crap into gold. You will have learned the art of bearing the Queen of the Dark's pressure, and you will have a diamond heart to show for it. Pearls, gold, diamonds; these gems are yours. You unearthed them, you polished them, you hand-cut every facet. Decorate your crown and string yourself a beautiful strand.

As you surf that edge between feeling it all fully and wallowing, between deciding you have had enough and numbing, the question arises, *What pain must be borne in order to learn from it and what pain can simply be avoided?* Your restrictive beliefs bring pain with them, so as you remake yourself, one belief at a time, you also stop attracting extra pain. Suffering and complaining are the norm in our world, so as you train yourself to cultivate the light and to nurture more happiness, you also resist sinking into collective suffering.

And yet, no matter how great your life gets—and please, get ready for it to get really, really great—there is a certain amount of death that will always be there to silhouette your bright life.

Get Ready for the Light As you come out of the underworld, before you can leave the dark for the dawn, before you learn the things and practice the practices that leave you feeling golden, there is a stop you need to make at the very center of your body. Before you can get to where you are going, you will need to commune with your inner knowing—your truth, your compass, your intuitive voice.

Your inner knowing carries messages from the other world, through you, into this world. It lives in the in-between. Your inner knowing can't wait to hear from you and get all parts of you back together again so you can remember who you truly are. So you can embody your genius.

I've always liked the time before dawn because there's no one around to remind me who I am supposed to be so it's easier to remember who I am.
BRIAN ANDREAS

Part Three

Embodying Your Genius

10

As Above, So Below
How a Goddess Pulls Herself Together

On a soul level, you are here to piece yourself together.
CAROLYN MYSS

few steps along this provocative path, you have now met Feminine
Genius and discovered how to align with her powerful energy.
You have learned how to navigate the waters of your personal
underworld, your dark. But before you splash fully into your light,
allow me to detain you for a few chapters. There is a particular energy
within your body that I want you to meet. Often misunderstood, it
is an energy that you, like most of us, have likely learned to fear, use
recklessly, or thrust into the shadow realm. As potent as fire, this
energy can burn you if you don't know how to handle it. And you may
indeed have been burned, perhaps painfully. Yet, it is an energy you
truly cannot live without.

Just as we humans learned to harness the awesome power of fire, so
too we can learn to harness this energy, the energy of Eros. Eros—sensual
love and desire—can help you retrieve your lost parts and refine your
inner guidance. Eros can help transform your confusion about your sexual
power into embodied confidence and wholeness. Eros can offer you intimate communion with the Beloved, whether in divine form as God or in
human form as another person, or—most importantly—as your own self.
Eros can blur the line between the sexual and the spiritual, and has the

power to bring heaven to meet Earth. Eros can help you become embodied and ensouled. Erotically empowered, you are destined to feel happy in your skin, spiritually authentic, fully expressed, and vibrantly alive.

To help you wrestle the brilliance of this energy back from the dream world of our collective psyche where it has been shut up for too long, let me offer you a fragment of a myth.

The goddess Isis is floating, adrift in a little boat in the River Styx, her hand trailing in the tourmaline water. She is heartbroken and near death because her beloved, Osiris—her flesh-and-blood lover and her metaphoric "other half"—has gone missing. Her trailing hand meets something in the water, and she pulls it up to get a better look. It is a leg, a human leg, with its foot still attached. Surprised, she reaches into the water again, and retrieves an arm, another leg, a torso, a head. She piles them in the boat with her, seeing them for what they are: the pieces of her beloved.

Isis keeps plunging her arm into the River Styx, that powerful waterway that, in death, helps all souls travel from this world to the other world. Trembling and triumphant, she drags the lost pieces of her beloved up from the depths and brings them home to her little boat. Isis *re-members* the disjointed limbs, organs, and appendages into an entire human body that is complete, shining, and whole. She reassembles her beloved who has been torn apart and cast into the underworld.

This complete and intact body looks achingly familiar, stirring something in her psyche. She is remembering what it feels like to have all her own once-fragmented parts reassembled as one glorious whole. She is remembering that the body of the beloved always wears the face of the Beloved. She is remembering that the Beloved also wears the face of the Goddess.

In this myth, Isis reminds: *Remember, you yourself are the Beloved.*

ISIS, MARY, AND THE VIRGIN: THE POWER OF GODDESS ARCHETYPES

If you haven't met her yet, the goddess Isis was one of the most important deities of ancient Egypt around 3,000 BC. Revered as the creatrix of all life, she was seen to wield the power of the Divine Mother and oversee the cycles of death and rebirth, creation and destruction, nature and magic. For many, Isis is one of the most familiar archetypes of empowered, complete, and sovereign femininity.

An archetype is a symbolic image or concept that is sourced from humanity's collective culture and psyche. A goddess, a fairy, a femme fatale—all are archetypes. However, our day-to-day lives have been nearly stripped of archetypes of women who are empowered, complete, and sovereign. As author Marian Wright Edelman puts it, "You can't be what you can't see." If you don't have models of empowered, complete, and sovereign women to look to, it is difficult to see yourself as powerful, whole, and free. By introducing you to the archetypes of the goddess Isis, Saint Mary Magdalene, and a virgin or two, I plan for you to get to see afresh some parts of yourself that may have been torn apart and cast into the underworld.

In the myth I just retold, the lover—and brother—of the goddess Isis is the god Osiris. As unusual as it may sound, the connection between Isis and Osiris is not incestuous. Rather, it's symbolic, a representation of the mystical union of opposites, of the masculine and feminine aspects of divine life-force energy uniting in one body. I see Isis's re-assembling of her beloved's body parts as her re-assembling her own self, the parts of her that sank into her own swampy shadow. In order to feel fully herself, and to honor the power of her body, she must re-member all parts—self and other, lover and beloved, sister and brother—inside herself. She can then see herself as the Beloved, the feminine flavor of God.

The joining together of a goddess and a god in this mystical symbolic union is sometimes called the sacred marriage, or *hieros gamos*. In the sacred marriage ritual, humans represent the deities. Through their sexual union, they merge the physical and spiritual worlds in an effort to spark the fertility that brings forth life. The sacred marriage is an important archetypal concept, whether or not it is consummated as an actual physical ritual. It is found not just in ancient Egypt with Isis and Osiris, but also cross-culturally in ancient Greece with Aphrodite and Adonis, in Hinduism with Shakti and Shiva, in Buddhism with Tara and Avalokitesvara.

As a concept (and as a practice), the sacred marriage recognizes Eros as a holy energy. It elevates Eros from a force that debases our humanity to a force that reunites us with divinity. In her book *Sacred Pleasure*, Riane Eisler confirms,

> The mystical or ecstatic state is said to provide those experiencing it a sense of indescribable inner peace, bliss, and even access to healing powers, along with a sense of unity or oneness with what mystics through the ages have called Divine Love. . . .There is strong evidence that sexual ecstasy was once also an important avenue to mystical or ecstatic states.[1]

Erotic energy, which is often assumed to prevent humans from knowing God, can actually allow mere mortals to embody mystical, divine love.

I see the existential drive of Eros as one that can balance the Divine Masculine and Feminine energies within you and can help you feel communion with the Divine within your earthly body. Whether experienced between you and God, you and another, or between you and you, erotic energy has the power to reveal sacred energy.

As a champion of sacred sexuality, Isis urges you to pull together the pieces of yourself that you may have cast aside because you couldn't fit them inside a downsized definition of *woman*. As an archetype, Isis urges you to remember that erotic energy is an essential part of the magic of birth, death, and rebirth. So that what is erotic need not be illicit, but can instead become devotional. So that you know your body is not only physically powerful but also metaphysically powerful. So that life need not be mundane, but can also become mystical. As in heaven, so on Earth. As above, so below.

oh, yes
you can have sex with soul

Mary Magdalene, the Saint

The archetype of Isis—at once a mortal and a deity, at once sexual and sacred—lives on in the more contemporary mythology of Saint Mary Magdalene. In case you don't know her well, Mary Magdalene is a figure from the Christian Bible, most known as a fallen woman, but also recognized as the thirteenth disciple, a spiritual companion of Jesus, and the first to see Christ rise from the dead. Some believe she is pictured in the painting *The Last Supper*. Isis was seen as a goddess from the get-go, but for Mary Magdalene, despite her canonization (or sainthood), it has taken the dominant culture several thousand years to recognize her as a true saint, not just as a repentant sinner.

I first encountered the connection between Isis and Mary Magdalene in Elizabeth Cunningham's book, *The Passion of Mary Magdalen*. Inspired by the apocryphal *Gospel of Mary*—Mary Magdalene's firsthand account of the story of Jesus Christ that was recovered in 1896—Cunningham asserts Mary's connection to Isis, and re-imagines Mary's life and her meeting with (and even marriage to) Jesus Christ.

But, hold on. Let me not get ahead of myself here. *Mary Magdalene's marriage to Jesus Christ?* Yes, indeed. In spite of her reputation as a whore, she is recognized by scholars Tom Kenyon and Judi Sion as a high priestess of hieros gamos and other erotic alchemical arts as passed down from followers of the goddess Isis. In their partially channeled book, *The Magdalen Manuscript: The Alchemies of Horus and the Sex Magic of Isis*, Kenyon and Sion offer the provocative idea that Mary Magdalene and Jesus Christ united in sacred marriage in part to fortify Christ's soul so that his body would be strong enough to embody his message and follow through with his work in the world.

Rather than a sidekick with questionable morality, as she has been portrayed for thousands of years, I see Mary as the leading lady in the story of Jesus Christ: his wife, companion, confidante, other half, and even tutor. Whether she was also, as I believe she was, an initiate in sex magic and the wife in sacred and literal marriage to Jesus Christ, we will likely never know for sure. After all, history is told by those with the pens with which to write it—or not write it—and they adjust it as they see fit.

Why I've asked Mary Magdalene to come make a cameo appearance in these pages is not only because she, like Isis, asks that the human body be held as sacred and that erotic energy be treated as holy, but also because Mary Magdalene asks us to remember that inner knowing—an intimate conversation with the Sacred—is possible on one's own without the middleman of established religion or convention.

It is important to note that the *Gospel of Mary* is part of the Gnostic gospels. Gnostics—another unruly band of mystical upstarts—generally believe in self-knowing. They believe that the answers to spiritual questions are to be found within ourselves, not outside ourselves. The word *gnostic* comes from the Greek word *gnosis*, meaning "knowledge," which is often used in Greek philosophy in a way that aligns with the English words *insight* and *enlightenment*. The archetype of Mary Magdalene asks us to remember that we don't need an intermediary to speak with the Holy One; we can strike up the conversation with our own little ol' mouths. She asks us to see that enlightenment—a direct realization that we are not (and never were) separate from the Divine—can be experienced through our own little ol' bodies.

Like the Gnostics did, Mary Magdalene asks you to view your physical body as materialized and concentrated soul. This is a radical departure from the tenets of asceticism, which were highly influential and pervasive at the time of early Christianity, and viewed the body—and especially the body of a woman—as sinful and impure. I see asceticism, the doctrine that says that you can reach elevated spiritual states through extreme self-denial, self-mortification, and pleasure-avoidance, reaching its tentacles into some aspects of modern culture and into some psyches of modern women. After all, for many of us, what are perfectionism and superwoman-itis if not attempts to reach elevated states through extreme self-denial, self-mortification, and pleasure-avoidance?

However, inspired by such a Gnostic as Mary Magdalene, you are invited to wake up and see that your corporeal impulses of erotic energy, desire, sensual delight, and pleasure can actually exalt your consciousness rather than limit it, can actually fortify your soul rather than tarnish it, and can actually light your modern, mystical path rather than obscure it. When you have lost the concept of yourself as the

Beloved, Mary Magdalene invites you to pull yourself together to again feel whole, a child of the Universe, and divinely at home in your body.

But Mary's is a radical invitation. After Isis's heyday and during Mary Magdalene's time, the culture at large had one lens through which to view a woman, a lens that we are still struggling with thousands of years later: that women are inherently inferior, unclean, sinful temptresses, and—unless carefully controlled—whores. The more sexually empowered the woman, the more likely she'd be designated a slut, and the less likely she'd be considered spiritually wholesome. Chances are that to some extent or another you too look at women and yourself through a (slightly more subtle) version of that lens—or struggle against being seen through that lens.

Most major world religions have been recorded, codified, and passed on mainly by men, and many do not hold women as physical or spiritual equals, with exceptions here and there in the more mystical branches such as Gnosticism, Kabbalah, Sufism, and Tantra. And collectively, our culture has taken so, so many pointers from the world's major religions. To this day, one of the biggest and most instantly effective slurs to a woman's value and trustworthiness is to accuse her of being a whore. And to this day, there is nothing like being called a whore to get your story discredited, distorted, and devalued. It is no wonder that you might find yourself conflicted about whether to embrace the power of your body or avoid it, to embody your sexuality or revile it, to directly know God in yourself or accept someone else's word for it. So, Mary Magdalene's story floats like a specter in our collective psyche.

However, only a couple of thousand years after the fact, Mary Magdalene is beginning to get her reputation back. In June 2016, the Catholic Church officially recognized July 22 as the feast day of Mary Magdalene and gave her the official title of Apostle of Apostles.

A woman, who believed that the body was a portal rather than an impediment to God, arm-in-arm with the Son of God? A woman, whose genius is the erotic, hooking up with the son of man? A woman, who presumed that it is natural to access the kingdom of heaven within, elevated as queen to the king of kings? A woman, who knew her way around the death/rebirth cycle, who may have taught our lord and savoir a thing or two? Whether actual history or powerful parable, it is pretty thought provoking, don't you think? You know what they say: behind every great man is a great woman. Or, as author Virginia Woolf put it, "I would venture to guess that Anon, who wrote so many poems without signing them, was often a woman."

Isis of ancient Egypt, Saint Mary Magdalene, and you, the modern goddess; each married sacredly to the Beloved and to herself. Radical, I know. But as one of my mentors, Regena Thomashauer, says, "A woman does not even begin to come alive until she is pressed up against the edge of what is radical for her." So here we are, sister, at the edge of radical.

Jump in with me.

The Temple Virgins

It would seem there are few words more damning for a woman than *whore*.

Certainly, the words *whore* and *prostitute*—two out of the impressive 220 words for a sexually promiscuous woman—have disparagement and damnation at their roots. The Old Norse *hora* means "adulteress"; the Middle English *hore* means "physical filth, slime, moral corruption, sin"; the Polish *nierządnica* means "disorderly woman"; and the Greek *porne* is related to *pernemi* and means "to sell" and likely referred to a female slave who was sold into prostitution. (Which compels me to ask, sold by whom, to whom? Morally corrupt according to whose rules? Promiscuous and disorderly by whose standards? Filthy and sinful as perceived through whose lens?)

But listen to this: way back in its English and Germanic roots, the word *whore* meant "one who desires." And if you trace back to other languages, in Latin, for example, *whore* is *carus*, which means "dear"; in Old Irish *cara* means "friend"; in Old Persian *kama* means "desire"; and in Old Sanskrit *kamah* means "love, desire." As you may know, the *Kama Sutra* is an ancient Hindu text on the philosophy of love, desire, and virtuous living, including poetry, sexual positions, and advice, named for the Hindu god of love, Kama.

So it would seem that the word *whore* has not always been entirely pejorative. In fact, it originally described a woman who was wise in the ways of love and desire, not bound by convention—perhaps even a minister of sacred marriage. As the standards of acceptability for women have changed, and as the divide between sexuality and spirituality has grown, so has the meaning of *whore*. We as women must write new endings to these fallible fables. We must take our remembering to the edge of radical. We can't wait two thousand years to have our sainthood confirmed.

No better women to help us with this than the temple priestesses and the virgins. The temple priestesses were young women who lived many thousands of years ago who got the opportunity to leave their homes before marriage and live in a temple and become masters of the arts of sex and love. It was understood that after a time serving in the temple, these young women would be considered "purified" for marriage.

Although they were experts in the erotic arts, the temple priestesses were considered to be virgins. The original meaning of the word *virgin* is "whole," as in, *complete unto to one's self*. As Marilyn Frye writes in her book, *Willful Virgin*, "The word 'virgin' did not originally mean a woman whose vagina was untouched by any penis, but a free woman, one not betrothed, not bound to, not possessed by any man. It meant a female who is sexually and hence socially her own person."[2] In contrast to how too many of us girls and women even today regard our bodies and our sexuality—as commodities to trade for love, acceptance, security, and belonging—the concept of the virgin temple priestess is quite striking.

Thousands of years ago, it was understood that if you were lucky enough to make love with a virgin or a temple priestess—like an Isis or a Mary Magdalene—you could hope to experience divine union and divine love. As Nancy Qualls-Corbett explains through her research and her book, *The Sacred Prostitute: Eternal Aspect of the Feminine*, the root cause of our present-day misunderstanding, confusion, and great suffering around sex is because we have lost the temple priestess and the virgin from our individual and collective psyche—the actual women themselves as well as the archetype of the erotically empowered, complete, and free woman that they represent. We must remember that sexual energy can be a vehicle for spiritual ecstasy, and that a woman's body, especially when held as sovereign and sacred, is particularly designed for this.

> Of course, women so empowered are dangerous.
> So we are taught to separate the erotic from most
> vital areas of our lives other than sex.
> **AUDRE LORDE**

Try this on for a moment. Put down the inherited lens you may have been looking at women through, and try on a new and different one. A lens though which someone like Isis, Mary Magdalene, or a temple priestess would have viewed women, as equal in value and in trustworthiness to men. You will begin to see that your enlightenment, your waking up, comes not through an arbiter, but through your direct self-knowing. And that feeling one with the Holy One is something you can do in your very body, not by leaving your body.

Refocus the lens and resist looking away, resist any discomfort, because what will come clear is this: the energy that we use to make babies, erotic energy, is the same energy that God uses to make life itself. Regardless of whether you choose to create new human life or not, it will start to become evident that erotic energy is the ultimate creative force, is the creative energy of life itself, and is thus the ultimate connection to the ultimate Creator.

Now, try this. While still looking through this radical lens, pan back a little and imagine a Feminine Genius walking around in her daily existence. You do not need to worry that she would suddenly become unable to hold down a job, change a diaper, be faithful to her partner, drive a car, tell a good joke, take the bar exam, do neurosurgery, write her novel, get to the meeting on time, keep a secret, meditate, or bring you soup when you have the flu. Just because she is at home in her body, in command of her erotic energy, and in communion with her voice, does not mean she is in danger of becoming untrustworthy, unsafe, a flake, or a prostitute. In fact, she is now in considerably *less* danger of selling herself out.

I know I just said a mouthful. Thirty mouthfuls. Thirty highly unorthodox mouthfuls. I just said that your erotic confidence can lead you to exalted consciousness. That erotic energy can reunite you with the natural magic of birth, death, and rebirth. That Eros can offer you greater strength, vitality, and integrity in your body so that you can walk your talk while you walk your path, so that you can fulfill your missions and follow your passions while here on Earth.

I just said that you *are* the Beloved. That pulling pieces of yourself out of the muck can help carve a path to your wholeness as a woman. That the more you feel whole, the more you can speak fluently with Eros. That you can make love with whomever, whatever, and however you call God. (And, no, this does in no way require you to enter into hieros gamos or become a member of the oldest profession, I promise).

I just said that not only can you walk hand in hand with God, but you can also speak with God yourself. No go-between needed, and we are talking speed dial. That you can feel erotically alive, spiritually alive, and virginal, all in the same body. And that you can wake up, here and now, in your body—and that you must.

If you jump into this upcoming section with me, and I hope you will, you will receive a sex re-education that I wish all women and girls could have received. You will learn why your body cannot lie, as well as an astounding reconfirmation of your body's intelligence. You will learn the language your body uses to communicate with you and why that language is the native tongue of your soul.

So, pull yourself together, goddess, and I will show you exactly where, in your wise body, is your direct line to the Divine.

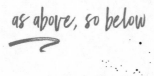

as above, so below

11

Sex Re-Education
The Birds and the Bees Get a Do-Over

Does my sexiness upset you?
Does it come as a surprise
That I dance like I've got diamonds
At the meeting of my thighs?
MAYA ANGELOU, "STILL I RISE"

What if what we have been taught about erotic energy, female sexuality, and the female body—and therefore, what we assume to be true—is all completely off the mark? As I see it, it is. So then, if I'm on to something here, a re-introduction to the birds and the bees just might be called for. If we are truly to trust Eros to exalt us rather than defile us, we all might require quite a profound re-education.

If our sexual education could get a do-over, women and men would honor and revere a woman's sexuality rather than objectifying and demeaning it. We women would feel confident in our bodies rather than feeling shame, confusion, deficiency, and vulnerability. We would embody what *we* feel is beautiful rather than what is *scripted* as beautiful. We would reconnect with our authentic sensuality rather than trying to appear sexy. We would wield our erotic power with consciousness and care, rather than use it to sell ourselves short and sell ourselves out.

If sexual education could get a makeover, we would glance back on history and marvel at the absurdity of a time when we made ourselves sick trying to become acceptable, lovable, marriageable, or fuckable. We would each reach into our own history and bring back into our adulthood what we felt as girls: that pleasure is as natural as breathing, that it is good to feel what we feel, and that it is safe to know what we know.

This is not the education most of us receive, but one we sorely need. So here goes.

I was four years old when the older neighbor boy convinced me to head off into the woods to play doctor. It was not a violent, physically harmful, or obviously psychologically damaging experience, as many girls' and young women's experiences are. The untrained eye would never know anything out of the ordinary had happened to me. But during my few visits with the "doctor," I became keenly aware that this was all about *his* exploration and enjoyment, not my own. I carried this belief—like so many women do—into my life and into my sexual identity until I was in my twenties: that in the realm of the erotic, *his* experience is more important than mine, and that my pleasure was at best incidental, at worst a distraction from the main event.

There are "official" sex ed experiences like classes, books with anatomically correct illustrations, or awkward conversations with awkward parents. And there are "unofficial" ones, such as my "doctor" experiences, "adult" magazines, internet pornography, dirty jokes, rumors relayed by older friends and siblings, even incest and outright sexual violence. Whether official or not, seen or not, our early education about sex and sexual energy indelibly shapes what we believe about ourselves, our bodies, our pleasure, our power, our safety, and our divinity, often for the rest of our lives.

I was thirteen years old during my first official sex ed class. I was uncomfortable and squeamish, like all the other girls and boys in the room. The intention of the class seemed to be to remove the mystery from this taboo topic and to help us make informed decisions about our bodies, the bodies of others, and our sexuality. We understood that it was our prepubescent duty to learn about sex, yet we also understood that sex was not something we should be doing or even thinking about in the first place. In the jail-like classroom with puce-colored walls, fluorescent lighting, and too-small desks, I stared at the pictures of male and female anatomy projected on the wall, trying to understand what fallopian tubes had to do with the way my body exploded into fireworks when I kissed a boy.

Many women have much more damaging introductions to sex and their bodies, as one of my online course participants, Violette, did. Perhaps you remember Violette from back in chapter 7. About thirty years after she'd been at the mercy of her father's belt, Violette shared with me what her formative sex education had been. She was told seven ways to Sunday—at home all through the week and during her father's evangelical Christian services—that as a woman, she was indisputably inferior to men. In fact, she was a walking profanity. Her very existence as a woman was blasphemous, obscene, and about as far from sacred as you could get. Inside and outside of church, Violette learned that her body, her desires, and her erotic energy were sinful and that her brightness and her enjoyment of her body had caused (and was currently causing) the downfall of humanity.

When Violette was twelve, her older sister, instead of taking her to the movies as promised, left Violette with a drug dealer friend. While her sister was gone, the man raped Violette and got her pregnant. Violette's family disowned her—the kind of disowned where she and her few belongings were tossed out into the night, the door of her home locked behind her. Terrified, Violette gave birth to her son alone in a dark alleyway, far away from her hometown, and far away from any sense of herself as okay.

Certainly, Violette's situation was extreme, yet what she learned to believe about her body, sexuality, and womanhood is more or less normal. Certainly not all Christians espouse the beliefs that affected Violette so deeply. And yet, regardless of our spiritual or religious upbringings, most of us have inherited these damning beliefs from the dominant culture, even if more subtly and less directly. I myself certainly have, even though I was raised as a kind of a new age, free-thinking, spiritual mutt. Certainly, there must be a better way to learn about our dear bodies.

Imagine with me for a moment if, instead of just fire and brimstone, Violette had been raised on Vedic Tantric philosophies. I know that I'm dreaming, that evangelical Christianity and Tantra are like the Bloods and the Crips who wouldn't be caught dead in the same 'hood. But humor me for a minute.

Tantra, as you may recall from part one, sees the energy of lifeforce—the power that animates all of life—as having a masculine aspect, called Shiva, and a feminine aspect, called Shakti. Through the lens of Tantra, the meeting, merging, and interplay of Shiva and Shakti is seen as the sacred, creative power of the Universe, whether inside you, between you and a partner, or in the world at large. Through the lens of Tantra, each woman's body is seen as a vessel for Shakti, as a flesh-and-blood embodiment of the Divine.

If Violette had been raised to see her body as a conduit for divine Shakti, she likely would not have spent a lifetime in physical and psychic stress, trying to divorce herself from her body, as she did. She likely would not spend most days in chronic physical and emotional pain, as she does now. Today, it is difficult for her to do her work and care for her son, and many of our Skype conversations happen with her in a hospital room or bed. Although she is still working to understand her mysterious illness and get better, she knows it is related to her early education about her body and erotic energy.

What if Violette had been taught she was precious and holy, as Tantrists teach that Shakti is to Shiva? What if every girl child saw her femininity as a set of strengths that she was thrilled to embody, and saw her sexual organs as a set of wonders that she was thrilled to own? Sadly, this is not even close to what most women and girls learn, and it certainly was not what my mentee Katya learned, either.

Katya wanted to learn to trust femininity within herself, other women, and the world, and to shift her painfully distorted views of her body, her sensuality, and her sexuality. Katya's mother, a cool and distant woman, was desperately disappointed that Katya had been born a girl rather than a boy. Katya shared with me a memory of herself at around two years old, ankles held up, bones crunched together, as her mother diapered her almost punitively, vocalizing disgust for Katya's female body parts.

As a child, Katya naturally delighted in things like eating, cuddling, cooking, the warmth of bathwater, and the slippery surprise of soap, but her mother labeled Katya's hunger for physical touch and life's pleasures as "lascivious." Until she was twelve, Katya tried to keep her masturbation a secret, but she developed chronic bladder infections that caused her to wet the bed. During a visit to the doctor, legs in stirrups, Katya heard her mother declare that Katya's infection was her punishment for being literally and figuratively dirty, and for doing "dirty stuff."

Katya grew to see her desires as shameful, and her body as something aberrant to be cured. She grew to understand that a lady's job was to get and keep total control over her sensuality and appetites, those "nasty bits" that could get her in trouble. No wonder Katya mistrusted anything to do with femininity. She showed up to my workshops anyway, sensing that having access to her feminine strengths within herself would shift everything.

I have to wonder how much more comfortable Katya would have been with her body if as a girl she and her mother had gone regularly to *yoni puja*, an ancient Tantric rite (that continues in present day) in which female body parts are worshipped. Again, I know I'm dreaming here, but what if Katya and her mother learned that *yoni*, the Sanskrit word for vagina, translates as "sacred gateway to life" and is considered to be the seat of the Divine? Tantrists believe that vaginal fluids originate in heaven, and that—à la hieros gamos—sexuality is a path to the holy union with the Holy One. Katya might have grown to assume that she was literally sitting on the throne of heaven.

During a yoni puja, Katya and her mother would have witnessed five liquids that represent earth, water, fire, air, and ether—yogurt, water, honey, milk, and edible oil—each poured consecutively over the yoni (either on the body of an actual woman or one made of clay). The liquids, having had direct and intimate contact with the living goddess, would then be considered purified and energized. They would then be collected in a vessel below the (real or clay) thighs, and consumed as a gift. Whether or not Katya and her mother would have imbibed, they would have learned that rather than a place of desecration, the yoni is a place of consecration. Katya would have learned that her femaleness was not something to cure, but in fact, something that can heal.

What if Katya and Violette—and all young men and women—learned about body parts and sex not just from the Tantrists but also from the Taoists of the 1700s? Author and activist Naomi Wolf, in her book *Vagina: A New Biography*, explains that Taoist men

> were trained in the classic sexual Yoga texts ("the
> education of the penis") to ensure that they sexually
> satisfied their wives and concubines with long foreplay
> and carefully timed thrusting, since personal and cosmic
> harmony, as well as healthy offspring, were all seen as
> being dependent on female sexual ecstasy.[1]

Through the eyes of the Tantrists and the Taoists, women's satisfaction and joy was once seen as vital, not incidental—a striking contrast to the "wham, bam, thank you, ma'am" concept that too many of us grew up with—and see all around us—as the norm.

WHAT DO WE WANT TO LEARN ABOUT SEX?

We are all, men and women alike, going to learn about sex, so the questions are: *What* will we learn? And how will what we learn shape how we treat our lovers and ourselves? And what will we pass along to future generations? It may be a lot to ask of a "tween" to comprehend Tantric and Taoist philosophies—although I would guess that learning affirming information about a woman's sexuality, value, and potential could be considerably less challenging than learning algebra. Regardless, I believe we would all be better off if we were exposed to philosophies such as these rather than be limited to the damaging ideas we currently receive through media, cultural norms, and social pressure.

For example, we live in an era when many, many people, including children and teenagers, have access to internet-enabled devices that connect easily to pornography. According to a *New York Times* article from January 2015, 93 percent of boys and 62 percent of girls have seen internet pornography. That includes porn that may feature rape, sexual violence, bondage, sex with children, incest, and bestiality.

Your Brain On Porn is a website that aggregates research and articles on the use and effects of pornography, reporting that young men as early as their teens are losing interest in "real" women because of the addictive nature of pornography and near-pornographic images in media. Their brains are not responding to the real thing, and in some cases, their relationships are suffering, and they are experiencing erectile dysfunction. For adults, there are websites and online forums where men (and women) can share their stories and get support as they "reboot" themselves from their self-proclaimed pornography addiction.

I know I'm stating the obvious by saying that for girls and boys, women and men alike, a realistic, positive sense of sexuality is hard to find in conventional culture. As writer Esther Perel puts it, "Magazine covers peddle smut while preaching sanctimony." The sex education that girls and women currently receive has us mistrust, vilify, exploit, and numb our sexuality almost instinctually, while at the same time, we groom ourselves to appear "sexy." We try to look good and play into what others seem to want, but we're not educated or empowered to have any actual ownership of our true sexuality.

A woman-positive sex re-education that honors and reveres female sexuality would make Keana's story extremely rare. Keana, a participant in my mentorship program, is a talented screenwriter and journalist. Daughter to second-generation Mexican Americans, she grew up in a working-class neighborhood of San Antonio, Texas. During her freshman year at one of the top liberal arts colleges in the country, there was a small gathering down the hall from her dorm room. When the group wanted food—which Keana had in abundance thanks to the care packages she would get from her grandfather—she invited them back to her room. While the rest of the party continued to booze it up in the common room, one guy shut Keana up in her bedroom and date raped her.

Keana was so paralyzed by what had been done to her that she didn't leave her dorm room for more than twenty-four hours. When she finally crept out to use the bathroom, she discovered that her nametag had been ripped off her door. A few months later, she attended a party hosted by one of the college's unauthorized, underground fraternities. There, in their common room, she found her nametag tacked up with dozens of others, all belonging to freshman women, and she realized that she had been one of many in an organized hazing ritual.

Keana's self-confidence nose-dived, and her grades plummeted. She eventually dropped out of her prestigious university and the future it promised, and spent the next twenty years plagued by self-doubt, writer's block, constant suicidal ideation, self-sabotage, a dependency on antianxiety medication, and an inability to enter any kind of stable, intimate relationship with a man.

A woman-positive, sex-positive re-education would make it harder to imagine disturbing scenarios like those from 2014 where fraternities from highly regarded American universities, such as Yale and Texas Tech, proudly and publicly countered the anti-rape slogans such as "No Means No" with "No Means Yes, and Yes Means Anal." We wouldn't have to ask the question that Vice President Joe Biden asked in June 2016, in his personal letter to the victim in the Stanford rape case, "Why did he think he had license to rape?" A woman-positive, sex-positive re-education would help ensure that young men such as these headline makers, who are destined to become our future partners, role models, policy makers, leaders, and fathers, would never even *imagine* such damage to—and disrespect of—women. They would not only value women implicitly, but would also know absolutely that such contempt hurts themselves as well.

As Violette learned, it is damaging to believe that your incarnation as a female caused the ruination of humanity and will continue to do so, one desire at a time, one vagina at a time. As Katya learned, it is traumatic to believe that your woman's body is a dirty, wicked problem that must be quarantined and sanitized. As Keana learned, it is ruinous to believe that as you walk through the world, your boundaries are a joke and your body is not your own. As I learned, it is depleting to believe that your pleasure is not something to honor and celebrate but something to hide or to fake.

As too many of us learn, it is disturbing to believe that we—and what we want—do not have a place here and that we would all be better off if only we could get very, very small. When the psychic, spiritual, and physical stress—caused by believing that our bodies and sexuality are toxic—abates, our "survival mode" (fighting, fleeing, freezing, "freaking out," compulsions, and addictions) can relax, and our birthright of emotional and physical "thriving mode" can return.

> Put away your pointless taboos and restrictions
> on sexual energy—rather help others to truly
> understand its wonder, and to channel it properly.
> **NEALE DONALD WALSCH,** *Conversations with God:*
> *An Uncommon Dialogue*

What if our education about sex actually delivered on its promise to help us make informed decisions about our bodies, the bodies of other people, and our sexuality, by empowering us to use this potent energy with intention and integrity? What if, instead of through contraband porn, gossip, church scandals, hazing practices, and dry sex ed classes, young women and men were taught by learned masters that sex is a high holy matter? What if we grew up assuming that, rather than being the cause of humanity's fall from divinity, every woman is an incarnation of the Divine?

What if, when walking down the street, instead of catcalls, women were routinely greeted with "Greetings, Goddess," as is customary in Tantric traditions, or "Hello, Empress," as in Rastafarian cultures? What if, along with Zen meditation techniques where you gaze into the flame of a fire, we were taught the yoni gazing techniques of ancient India and Japan, which persist today, as just as viable a way to calm the mind and call in the Holy One?

What if we grew up assuming all women have a *sacred gateway to life* between our thighs, that our sex energy purifies rather than dirties, that we are sacred vessels rather than sex objects, that our pleasure is a priority, and that both our *"Hell, yes!"* and our *"Fuck, no!"* will be respected? What might be different if we—Violette, Katya, Keana, you, and me—all learned this from the start? The ripple effects would be *profound*. Remember that long-lost, sorely missed, goddess-inclusive era I mentioned a while back? Bring it on.

SEXUAL *AND* SPIRITUAL

In order to revive that long-lost, inclusive era, we have to throw out the assumption that spirituality and sexuality, two of our essentially human drives, are at opposite ends of our spectrum of values. Conventionally, spiritual energy is designated pure and virtuous, the holy North Pole, while sexual energy is deemed dirty and dangerous, the shadowy South Pole. So it can be a shock for some people to entertain the idea that erotic energy and sacred energy might share a zip code, and that Eros could be one of the faces of God.

But it was not always so. Author and anthropologist Riane Eisler states that for our prehistoric ancestors, "there was not the distinction between nature and spirituality, between the religious (or sacred) and our day-to-day lives (including our sex lives)."[2] She goes on to say that "in sharp contrast to much of later religious imagery and dogma, which often sacralizes suffering and pain, our ancestors sacralized pleasure, particularly that most intense physical pleasure we are given to feel: the pleasure of sexual ecstasy."[3] It turns out, the divide between the sexual and the sacred is *inherited*, not *inherent*.

Yes, sexual energy is like fire. Fire is powerful. Potent. Primal. One of the keys to our evolution as humankind. Just like fire can be a destructive force if used without care and awareness, so can sex and sexuality. The culturally accepted idea is that if we play with the fire of eroticism, we will burn down the house, the village, the civilization. Our evolved human status will go up in an inferno of passion. Truly, sexual energy can often bring with it mighty sensations and emotions. It can be unpredictable. Eros is primal. It resists domestication, hasn't read etiquette books, and prefers the laws of nature to the rules of humans.

Yet even though life-force energy is indeed some of the most potent stuff there is, it is not innately destructive. Some would say that it is the *nature* of erotic energy to spawn horrors like violent internet pornography, date rape, rape culture, sexual slavery, child prostitution, genital mutilation, and incest. I would say that it is not the *nature* of sexual energy to create and perpetuate these horrors; it is our *misunderstanding* and *gross misuses* of sexual energy that can create and perpetuate these horrors.

Certainly, we need to understand the potential dangers that go along with following a sexual desire so we can make informed decisions. Certainly, sex can lead to pregnancy, emotional attachment, or sexually transmitted infections. But the energy itself isn't dangerous. Like fire, a knife, anger, or hunger, sexual energy is a source of power and a potent tool.

And, just as fire has been key to our evolution as human beings, "human sexuality is not a hindrance but rather a help in the human quest for higher consciousness,"[4] as Riane Eisler says. As we strive to develop as awake, aware, spiritual beings, we must, instead of restraining and abstaining from erotic energy, seek to understand and harness it, as we have sought to understand and harness the power of fire.

A true sexual re-education requires us to become masterful at, empowered by, and literate in one of life's most potent energies. Instead of being afraid of Eros's strength and magnitude, we must become students of it. As Riane Eisler says:

> This is basically what the modern revolution of
> consciousness is about: the gradual deconstruction
> and reconstruction of the stories and images that have
> for so long served to mold our minds, bodies, and
> souls to fit the requirements of a system driven by
> punishment, fear, and pain.[5]

Our sexuality need not savage us; it can set us free. We need not regress; we can advance.

> Your whole idea about yourself and your
> beauty is borrowed—borrowed from those
> who have no idea of who they are themselves
> and have not seen their own beauty.
> OSHO

This kind of sex re-education can help you to notice that the urges of your body aren't inherently sinful or wanton. In fact, your hunger is holy. That you can rock your unique brand of beauty, whether or not it even vaguely resembles what's on the billboard at the mall. That you can know—as you did at some point in your girlhood—that it is good to feel good and that you can love what you love. This kind of sex re-education comes directly from the offices of Feminine Genius.

This kind of sex re-education doesn't mean you must look and act obviously sexual all the time. Sexual energy is simply life-force energy. Eros is simply the sensual experience of being alive.

This kind of sex re-education helps you realize that erotic energy comes in mild, medium, and spicy versions. It only looks like what we know as sexual energy in its full-blown, spicy versions. Mild, for example, could be a sense of sensual aliveness, of tasting, seeing, hearing, smelling, touching, and intuiting with greater subtlety and intensity. Medium could show up as flirtation, fortitude, or calculated risk-taking. Spicy could be more obviously erotic, including states of sexual turn-on, arousal, ecstasy, bliss, and orgasm.

This kind of sex re-education reminds you that it is your prerogative to take pleasure in your body and womanhood. In your daily life, it is possible that you will be the only one who knows that what is actually pumping through your veins is sensual energy. Everyone else might just notice the rare sight of a woman who is comfortable in her own skin and enjoying herself, just as she is. A woman who trusts and admires her feminine strengths, and presumes everyone else does, too. A woman who refuses to apologize for herself, for her body, or for taking up space.

This Feminine Genius loves that her life and her pleasure are her own again. She feels a part of life, as if she belongs by default. She is no longer trying to be someone else, and in her presence, you feel more like yourself (and you like yourself more). Her lifelong undercurrent of anxiety and stress has been replaced by her bone-deep well-being—the flood of gratitude from one who knows she has chosen her life, and she has chosen well. If you ask her, she will tell you her life is far from perfect, and often quite brutally painful, but that she no longer feels lost. She will tell you that it feels satisfying to be in daily conversation with something at once greater than herself yet something so simply herself.

This Feminine Genius will tell you that these interior treasures can be taken by no one. She will tell you that whatever she had to invest, go through, let go of, lose, or humbly laugh into being, whatever she had to learn or unlearn, was all worth it. A thousand, thousand times over, dear goddess, worth it.

And she would wish the same for you.

I know you don't see many women embodying this. Not very many women know that this is their birthright. But given the right lens through which to be seen and to see herself, this potential is in every woman. Every woman, without exception. Instead of feeling like a walking profanity, a woman who embodies this potential feels *just right*. After all, *profane* is a descriptor for that which has been cast out of the temple and is no longer sacred. For a moment, gaze at yourself with re-educated eyes and notice that not only have you been unjustly cast out of the temple, but that you *are* the temple.

what if you knew your body as a living, breathing, feeling temple of the Divine Feminine?

Then together we can make the journey home. We can make the journey from castoffs to vessels of sacred wisdom, from walking profanities to walking shrines to the Divine. *Profound* means "that which reveals vast, deep, divine insight." When a woman sees herself, and demands to be seen by the world, not as *profane* but as *profound*, all our healing can finally begin.

Woman: a profound body of knowledge well worth learning well

12

An Oracle of One's Own
Your Direct Line to the Divine

The number of steps from you to God is zero.
NATHAN OTTO

Every word on every page has been leading you here.

The confidence, guidance, and salvation you hoped to find *out there*, can be found *in here*, within your body beautiful. Eros can embolden and impassion you for the life you are here to live. The wellspring of your light, fire, and inner knowing—the headquarters of your Feminine Genius—I call your Oracle. Actually, I call it the Oracle Between Your Thighs.

But let's back up a bit.

Let me tell you a creation story of when the Divine created human beings. When she (we'll call her she, shall we?) was done making the multitudes, she was tired and wanted to take a break. But we humans, fruitfully multiplying, wouldn't give her a rest. We humans had questions. We wanted divine guidance; we wanted answers to our conundrums about what to do with our lives: how many children to have, or whether to have them at all, who was our best partner, the right way to pray, whether or not to drink water with our meals, whether to set up our doors to the east or the north, and so on.

The Divine took off to the highest mountaintop, sure she'd get her well-deserved break, but of course we humans found her there.

We named her *Oracle* and gave her the official job description of *wise counsel, divine wisdom,* and *spiritual authority.* Beyond exhausted, she went into the deepest cave she could find, but of course, we found her there as well. Finally, she took off to the Bahamas, but of course we found her there as well, even behind her oversized rock star sunglasses.

So then the Divine formulated the perfect plan: she broke herself up in a zillion little pieces and placed one piece inside each human being because she knew that was the last place we would ever think to look, and at last she'd get some peace. Her plan has worked brilliantly ever since.

I was fifteen when I heard this story from one of my most inspiring dance teachers. For me, it served as an inflection point, one that you, beloved, have already crossed over, simply by having read this far. From this point forward, you will always remember that what you are aching for cannot be found *out there,* not in parental wisdom, in papal wisdom, in magazine wisdom, or even best friend wisdom. It can only be sourced from within. Your own inner knowing can be clarified, catalyzed, and inspired from your trusted sources *out there,* but its source is within you.

So would you like to know exactly where within you this power source *is?* Let me introduce you to your own personal Oracle.

The word *oracle* has its roots in the Latin word *orare,* "to speak or to pray." Any oracle is a bit like an orator, as in a speaker, debater, lecturer, or sermon giver. In past times and cultures, an oracle was understood to be a physical person (although sometimes it was a location like a spring or grove, or an object like a shrine or temple) that not only had the ear of God but was also the mouthpiece of God.

Just as in many religious and spiritual traditions, folks believed that you couldn't speak directly to God yourself, but that you could connect through an oracle. If you had a question for the omnipotent and omniscient Divine about what you should do with your life, how you should behave or think, you would go consult the oracle, which was endowed with the powers of prophecy. It could see the future and know what was best for you. The oracle's guidance, officially stamped with the seal of the Sacred, was safe to put into action.

The Oracle as direct line to
The Divine—YES
That it is outside of you—NO

Your own personal Oracle is within you. It is right where the Divine placed it so reverently and irreverently, right at your South Pole, in every wise cell of your naughty bits. On the coattails of the Gnostics, I say that your Oracle isn't out there on the highest mount. You don't need a go-between. You've got your very own Oracle, factory-installed in your sexy, wise woman's body. You won't find her in the depths of a cave, on the highest mountaintop, or in the Bahamas. She is in you. In your body. In your female reproductive organs, in fact, all nestled nicely in the cauldron of your pelvis.

you can know
Truly, who can know, but you?

AN ANATOMY OF YOUR ORACLE

Let me offer an even deeper view into why I believe that your *inner knowing*—intelligent, intuitive, divine guidance—can be found in your pelvis, your sexual center. The geographic area of your Oracle, below your belly button and above your tailbone, is also known as your pelvic bowl, and holds most (but not all) of your female sexual organs, specifically your vulva, vagina, clitoris, uterus, ovaries, and pelvic nerve. These lovely bits distinguish you as female and endow you with physical and metaphysical female superpowers.

Your pelvic bowl is made up of the bones at the base of your spine, your sacrum and pelvis. If you reached around and massaged your lowest low back (go ahead, you know you want to), you would feel the bones that make up your sacrum. The Latin root of *sacrum* means "sacred," by the way. The ancient Romans called the sacrum *os sacrum*, meaning "holy bone." The ancient Greeks called it *hieron osteon*, meaning "temple or sacred place." Ancient Egyptians also assumed the sacrum to be the seat of special power.

If you then placed your hands on your low belly and inched your fingers downward (go ahead, it won't bite), the next bony protrusion you would find would be your pelvic bone, part of your pelvis. The word *pelvis* comes from Latin and means "a cup, bowl, or vessel." *Sacred vessel.* A much better name than those our sexual organs often get called, if you ask me. And nice to know that at one point, it was built into our language that you have serious sacredness *down there*, not just something mundane or profane.

So, there you have it. Your female reproductive organs are holy. And you are the proud owner of an Oracle, a sacred vessel for new life, ideas, desires, visions, and passions.

HOW YOUR ORACLE KNOWS

Let me offer an even deeper view into how your Oracle relays your inner knowing to you. As practitioners of Traditional Chinese Medicine and acupuncture can tell you, the organs of the body such as the liver, kidneys, and spleen each have a distinct and measurable pulse. And, at least one of your sex organs does as well.

There is an unusual medical instrument with a decidedly unsexy name—the vaginal photometer (I told you, not sexy)—that uses light waves to measure the pulsations inside the human vagina. And the pulse that it measures is a different and distinct one from the pulse of your heart and blood. And guess when the pulse of your vagina increases in intensity or speed? Not necessarily during sexual arousal or orgasm, although it can then, too, but when you are emotionally moved, inspired, and impassioned.

Your flesh-and-blood vagina pulses distinctly and measurably when you are experiencing a surge of meaning, love, euphoria, anticipation, gratitude, or pride. Your lady parts have a pulse, which a scientific instrument can detect and gauge, that fluctuates when you feel deeply connected, intensely alive, and divinely motivated. Your vagina *knows*.

And so does your clitoris. The singular biological function of your lovely, pearly clitoris is to create sensual pleasure—for you! All female mammals (and a few other species) have such an organ, one that never ages, sags, or atrophies. Your human clitoris has 8,000 nerve endings. The average penis has half that number, only 4,000. Your clitoris is somewhere between the size of a pea and a grape, yet has twice the capacity for pleasure than the considerably larger, banana-sized male member. When it comes to nerve endings and pleasure potential, peas beat bananas two-to-one, every time.

Bottom line? Your body was biologically designed to experience pleasure. Twice as much than the average dude. Whoever or whatever designed the human body blueprinted into your flesh and blood a structure devoted entirely to your pleasure.

It also built into your biology a remarkable link between your pleasure and your confidence. When you experience (or expect to experience) states of pleasure (whether the mild, medium, or spicy kind), the nerve endings in your pelvis fire off. Those pleasurable sensations are relayed through your pelvic nerve, to your spinal cord, and up to your brain, which then releases dopamine, a neurotransmitter. Now, dopamine, sister, equals *confidence*. Neuroscientists tell us that dopamine is critical for motivation and desire. If dopamine is depleted or blocked, you may lose the will to strive, even the ability to move.

The good news is that you don't need any scientific devices to measure any of this. You may have not yet noticed the knowing pulses in your vagina, or that when your pleasure increases, so does your confidence. But if you take a few moments to turn your attention to your nether region, you can feel it for yourself.

There in your pelvis is the location of your knowing, your clarity, your confidence, your full-body *yes*. There is the seat of your Oracle. What are you truly passionate about? What is your purpose? What is meaningful to you? What moves you? What are your favored forms of self-expression? Why are you here? What is your calling, your mission, your contribution; and will you be able to pull it off? What do you want? And how can you trust what you hear? The pulses in your vagina *know*. The confidence instigated by your clitoris *knows*. Your sexual, sensual, erotic life-force energies *know*. Your Oracle *knows*.

Author Naomi Wolf discovered that the female brain and the vagina, rather than being two distinct organs of *knowing*, are more like a single system—a system in which a woman's sexual history, life experiences, and beliefs about her femininity can affect the functioning of her body, mind, and soul. In *Vagina: A New Biography*, which draws on the findings of numerous neuroscientists, Wolf suggests that cultures that practice female genital mutilation and rape as a tactic of war do so in part to affect a woman's thinking, sense of self, agency, and her "inner light." Wolf also shares research that shows that some somatic conditions that at first seem unrelated to sexual energy—like vertigo, ringing in the ears, low physical stamina, and a muscular issue that causes a woman to have unusually poor balance—are dramatically more present in women who have sexual abuse or rape in their histories.

It becomes even more understandable why we women, more often than not, have developed a confusing relationship with our bodies, erotic energy, sex organs, wants, desires, and passions. Statistics confirm that about one-third of us have been profoundly or violently wounded in these areas. It is as though one of our legs has been cut off, and we wonder why it is so hard to run to catch the bus. We have ignored, dumbed down, or excised entirely our sensual and somatic superpowers, and we need these amputated parts of ourselves back. Hello, Oracle.

As Naomi Wolf concludes, "To understand the vagina properly is to realize that it is not only coextensive with the female brain, but is also, essentially, part of the female soul . . . a mediator and protector of women's highest, most joyful, and most unbroken sense of self."[1] Your Oracle (which includes not only your vagina but also all the sexual reproductive organs in your pelvis) is not separate from your brain, it is in partnership with your brain. Your Oracle not only channels your erotic energy, it also channels your soul. Your Oracle not only creates life, it also brings meaning to your life. Your Oracle is not only an organ of pleasure, but also an organ of truth. Your Oracle, it turns out, is not an appendage that you tow around like a dinghy on a ship, but an engine, steering wheel, compass, and headquarters, all in one.

After a period of sexual awakening or after a singular incredible sexual experience, women often feel surges of unapologetic creativity and self-expression. A positive, full-body sensual experience lights a woman up and brings all of her on line. Perhaps you have experienced this yourself, when ecstatic erotic experiences can create a deeper sense of meaning and connection between you, other people, and life. When this channel of your power is once again flowing, in its mild, medium, and spicy forms—Watch. Out. World.

But why *here*, you might ask. Why not in your brain, why not in your heart, why not in your gut, why not in your big toe for that matter? Why do I insist on opening up a can of worms by insisting that the power and wisdom of your Oracle is rooted in your pelvis?

THE PASSIONATE PELVIS

Remember Riya? The woman in chapter 3 who learned, in the backseat of her family car when she was a wee four years old, to button up her enthusiasm for life? When I first met Riya, she shared a recent experience of relocating her passion, her passion for life and for her work, as well as for her sensual life with her husband. In a Skype session and with guidance from one of her spiritual mentors, Riya put on, ironically enough, Peter Gabriel's "Passion," from the soundtrack of the movie *The Last Temptation of Christ*, and began an improvised dance meditation to access her primal energy and passion. As instructed, she dropped her awareness into her pelvis and low belly and moved from there.

pelvis. low belly. move.

Riya moved. She danced; she undulated her whole body; she swiveled her hips and embodied the music. She went for it. She growled. She roared. She wept tears of sadness for having kept down her primal yet innocent energy. And she laughed, feeling, as she put it, like a divine child.

Something bubbled up that she hadn't felt in years. Riya felt sexy, she felt wild, she felt whole, and she felt beautiful. It was the first time in maybe her whole life that she felt *present*. As she rested after the sweaty session, she reflected that she had reconnected to her innate untamed essence—her passion—feelings she remembered having as a child.

In the days and weeks after her dance of passion, Riya began to hear clearly her own inner voice. And then she and I met, rolled up our sleeves, and got to work. Through our conversations in our coaching sessions and through movement and meditation practices at our retreats, Riya updated her restrictive beliefs about her body. Seeing her body for the first time as a temple helped her prioritize healthful eating and exercise for the first time in her life. As Riya got "back in her body," she was able to get back on speaking terms with the same wants, passions, and desires she had buried as a young child. Riya practiced letting her passion direct her in her daily life, in her work in the world, and—slowly, but surely—into a more fun and rich connection with her husband.

Riya took it on faith that she would be able to re-access her passion and inner guidance through her pelvis and low belly region, the place in her body that her erotic energy sourced from. She was instinctively drawing on the power of *kundalini*, an energetic force coiled in the pelvic region that ancient traditions recognize as the wellspring of our passion, power, confidence, inspiration, creativity, and knowing.

The Power of Kundalini

Please welcome kundalini. Kundalini is a form of energy. It is primal energy, life-force energy, the energy of Shakti. The term *kundalini* is derived from the Sanskrit word *kundal*, meaning "coiled," and is described in the Upanishads as well as Vedic and Tantric texts as early as the sixth century. Your kundalini—or Shakti—energy is considered to be spiraled like a potent snake or sleeping goddess at the base of your spine, in your sacrum, at the "root" of your body, waiting to be awakened.

Many of those who work with kundalini energy see it as libidinal and instinctive, as well as spiritual. Some look at kundalini energy as a biological mechanism that links the activity of the reproductive system and the brain. Kundalini is considered to be *in-dwelling*, meaning it is only accessed *through* your body.

Some go so far as to say that kundalini is an evolutionary impulse that can guide human beings toward greater consciousness and enlightenment, and that it has been referred to directly by many founders of major faiths, including Christ, Buddha, and Muhammad. (And let's not forget the goddess Isis and Saint Mary Magdalene, too.) Some scholars say that energies like the *spirit* in "Holy Spirit," the *kingdom* of the "kingdom of God within," and the *light* of enlightenment are all other names for kundalini.

Kundalini energy practices are designed, through breath, movement, and meditation, to release the erotic, creative, potential energy that originates in your pelvis. Through breath, movement, and meditation, it then moves up your spine and throughout your whole body, so you can have access to your innate radiance, well-being, peace, and vibrancy—your passion.

As I see it, your Oracle, in your passionate pelvis, is the seat of your physical and metaphysical female superpowers. Your Oracle helps to define your femaleness and to source your life-force energy, whether called kundalini, Shakti, Holy Spirit, or Eros.

Physically, your Oracle is the grouping of female reproductive organs that live in your pelvis, below your belly button and above your tailbone, whose functions include (but aren't limited to) producing and regulating hormones, conducting experiences of pleasure, as well as synthesizing the raw biochemical ingredients needed to create and incubate new life.

Metaphysically, your Oracle is where the sacred and the sexual meet. Your Oracle is where the other world and this world meet. Your Oracle is where your soul and your soma meet. Your Oracle is a great determinant of whether you, like a source of light and fire, are turned *on* or *off*. It is through your Oracle that your deepest wisdom bubbles up, like a celebratory bottle of champagne. Your Oracle knows what brings you joy, fulfillment, confidence, clarity, meaning, and pleasure, and what does not. She is the seat of your "Hell, yes!" and your "For heaven's sake, no!" Business, book, or baby, are all born here. Although possibly paradoxical, the physical and metaphysical functions of your Oracle are both true.

So, instead of consulting an external oracle, let's have you awaken your own Oracle. Let's start gently, as I realize it might be a shock to the system to simply strike up a conversation with your pelvis.

ORACLE PRACTICE #1   ORACLE MEDITATION

This Oracle meditation is designed to wake up a slumbering Oracle. It is a wake-up call, but not like that obnoxious, police siren type of alarm clock that shocks you out of slumber; more like a gentle Zen kind of clock that slowly fills the room with light and seduces you awake.

The Oracle meditation is a sassy twist on the traditional Buddhist Vipassana contemplative mindfulness meditation practice, which is designed to help you focus your awareness on a specific part of your body and keenly observe the sensations present there. Like any meditation, it is designed to help you choose deliberately what to focus on. In this case, for example, rather than focusing your awareness on your endless to-do list, you will direct your awareness to the source of your power instead.

1   Sit or stand comfortably and place your hands on your low belly, your Oracle.

2   While you would usually be aware of drawing your breath in and out of your nose or mouth, imagine

instead drawing your breath *in* through the base of your spine and *out* the top of your head.

3 As you draw your breath in, imagine it waking up, turning on, nourishing, soothing, or enlivening your Oracle—the lovely and lively spot on your body that rests below your belly button and above your tailbone.

4 As you breathe out, imagine your breath shooting out the top of your head and cascading in front of you like a waterfall.

5 Continue this "circular waterfall breathing," as I call it, imagining each in-breath as a cool breeze or a warm caress, continuing to wake up, turn on, nourish, soothe, or enliven your Oracle.

6 Notice what sensations and emotions come up as you place your awareness on your Oracle in this way. If thoughts, beliefs, judgments, pulsations, or preferences also come up, simply observe them, thank them for sharing, and let them pass on just as they came.

That's it. A simple (but kind of saucy) meditation practice, ideal for reacquainting you with your Oracle. Simply and kindly placing your awareness on something (especially when that something has been a little or a lot out of your awareness) is the first step to any profound change.

> There is more wisdom in your body than in your deepest philosophies.
> **FRIEDRICH NIETZSCHE,** *Thus Spoke Zarathustra*

Your Oracle is a guidance system reconnecting you to the wisdom of your body and the intelligence of your soul. As you practice, your Oracle can help you make daily choices and determine crucial next steps, even if you have felt disconnected from and doubtful about your wisdom up until now.

Over eight years ago, Safya sought me out to help her gain clarity on whether or not to leave her marriage. Disconnected from and doubtful about her wisdom, Safya had literally made herself sick trying to decide. She wasn't sleeping, and much of the time she was nauseated and anxious. Self-doubt was her constant companion. While she wanted to find clarity for her current situation, we both knew that she also needed a way to find clarity for *any* situation, now and going forward.

In our private sessions, we started to explore what she really wanted for herself and for her life. At first, Safya couldn't come up with any answers. She felt disturbed that she was clear about what other people wanted for her and for her life, but that she herself just didn't really know. She didn't even know how to know.

Over the past eight years, Safya learned how to know and has frankly *mastered* how to know. She first needed to learn the language of her body's wisdom, which is as refined, systematic, and complete as any verbal language and has allowed Safya to think less, yet know more. Her inner knowing has guided her to leave that marriage, get into a whirlwind five-year romance with a wealthy celebrity, get over devastating heartbreak, build her business to remarkable profitability, and have her first child with a much younger man. It hasn't always felt easy for her, but it has always felt true.

Let me share with you a version of what I did with Safya so many years ago, so that when you ask what it is you truly, madly, deeply want, you can access your body's wisdom as well as trust the answers you hear. Let's get you started with the ABCs of your Oracle's language: your *yes* and your *no*.

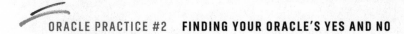

ORACLE PRACTICE #2 FINDING YOUR ORACLE'S YES AND NO

1 Take a moment to get quiet and perhaps close your eyes. I suggest putting your hands on your low belly, your Oracle.

2 Begin by taking a few breaths that are slower and more deliberate than usual. Direct your awareness to your breath on the inside of your body, waking up and nourishing the inside of your body, almost like a massage or a caress.

3 Now, please ask yourself a series of four questions to which you *know* your answer is *yes*.
   - "Is my name (your name)?"
   - "Do I love (someone you love)?"
   - "Do I enjoy (something you enjoy, perhaps a scent, taste, or touch)?"
   - "Do I feel vibrantly alive when I (something that brings you alive)?"

4 After answering each of the questions, bring your awareness to your Oracle (specifically to your low belly, the area under your hands) and notice what *sensations* and *emotions* you feel, and where you feel them.

5 Notice the common thread between the sensations and emotions you noticed in all four *yes* answers. This is how your Oracle says *yes*.

6 Now, please ask yourself a series of four questions to which you know your answer is *no*.
   - "Is my name (someone else's name)?"
   - "Do I love (someone you abhor or find, well, extremely challenging)?"

- "Do I enjoy (something you detest, perhaps a scent, taste, or touch)?"
- "Do I feel vibrantly alive when I (something that saps your will to live)?"

7   After answering each question, bring your awareness to your Oracle (specifically to your low belly, the area under your hands) and notice what *sensations* and *emotions* you feel, and where you feel them.

8   Notice the common thread between the sensations and emotions you noticed in all four *no* answers. This is how your Oracle says *no*.

How to use this? I suggest you start by asking your Oracle, on a daily basis, what I refer to as "low stakes" questions such as, "Wear this skirt or these pants?" "Peaches or guavas?" "Coffee or tea—or water?" "Make a detour into that store?" "Say that awkward thing now?" "Stay in tonight or go out?" and follow the *yes*es and *no*s that you sense. Then work your way up to higher-stakes questions like, "Should I get married to him?" "Should I have a baby?" "Should I stay or should I go?" or "Should I start this business or that one?"

Practice first with low-stakes questions to increase your confidence so that later you can use this with more complex queries in your life. I will say it again: start with low stakes. Don't start out with biggies. Take some time to experiment with questions that won't really affect much of anything in your life, whatever you choose. I know sometimes it feels like life or death to choose between the skirt and the pants, but it is not. Whether to terminate a pregnancy or not, whether to take your father off life-support or not, that is literally life or death. Work up to high-stakes questions like those.

There is no one right way your Oracle's *yes* and *no* should feel. It is different from woman to woman, but here are some feelings that clients and course participants have reported over the years that I have offered this practice:

> *Yes* **feels like:** Expansion and moving toward something;
> light, easy, and free, like air can move through me;
> powerful and happy; a horizontal opening starting
> in my belly; a softening smile; alive yet peaceful and
> calm swirling sensations; a tingling thrill in my heart
> and pelvis; positive, expansive, and relaxed; tingles
> throughout my body; warmth in my vagina; not exactly
> arousal, but kind of; a feeling of joy, bliss, and buzzing;
> assurance, like standing my ground.

> *No* **feels like:** Contraction and moving away from
> something; a tightness in my shoulders and upper back;
> like shrinking back into my spine; tightening in my
> throat; a warning cringe in my gut; constriction and
> panic in my belly; a flush of anger; retreating inside;
> wrongness with tight muscles; deadening dullness;
> pushing away; uncertainty, closure, and guardedness;
> my mind and thinking gets over-active.

There is no one right response to discovering your Oracle's *yes* and *no*, and there is no one right way to use this tool, but here are some more reports from women clients and course participants on what it is like for them:

> **Discovering my Oracle's** *yes* **and** *no* **is:** Such a great
> blessing to be able to read my body's language and know
> my real answer even before mentally assessing; in all
> honesty, partly terrifying, partly mesmerizing; now I don't
> need a pendulum or muscle testing; an embodied way to
> improve my happiness and my decision-making skills;

a powerful guide to help me understand what might
be going on when I feel triggered or reactive; and, an
extremely valuable tool to stop second-guessing myself.

By learning your Oracle's *yes* and *no*, you are learning your Feminine
Genius ABCs. Brava! (And, just like learning any new language, it
will get richer and more nuanced as you go. A bit later, I will show
you how these ABCs become a full language of words, sentences, and
paragraphs; even sonnets, odes, bulleted instruction lists, slam poetry
pieces, and full-scale rapturous visions.)

The first song my son learned was "Twinkle, Twinkle, Little Star."
He would sing it, pulling himself up by the railings of his crib, often
saying "la, la, la, la," in place of any words. It was cuteness overload.
The second song my son learned was the ABC song, and I noticed then
that the two songs actually have the same melody. Your ABCs, as sung
to you from your body beautiful, are just like little stars.

Listen. Look. Those little twinklers are re-assembling into your new
North Star.

And never was there a more wondrous compass than your Oracle.

> You think you need a map,
> but what you really want is a compass.
> **SETH GODIN**

13

Trusting Your Oracle

Distinguishing the Voices of Doubt, Delusion, Reason, and Intuition

There is deep wisdom within our very flesh,
if we can only come to our senses and feel it.
ELIZABETH A. BEHNKE

So, you've got your Oracle. Your very own direct line to the Divine. Woman, this is great news indeed! You have located your soul's mouthpiece, and you have started the conversation flowing. Now it's time to find out all that your inner knowing wants you to know. It's time to use your Oracle as engine, steering wheel, captain's quarters, and compass. Let the good times roll!

And yet.

Over the years, as I have been reintroducing women to their Oracles and inner knowing in this way, one of the first doubts I often hear is something like, "Having an Oracle between my thighs sounds good and all, but why just this one little spot? Why not listen to my whole body, if it's as wise and trustworthy as you say it is?"

Oh, yes, your whole body *is* infinitely wise. Of course there are other places and types of intelligence throughout it, including (but not limited to) your head, heart, and gut. I am sure you are used to hearing "be rational," "listen to your heart," and "trust your gut instinct." Yet, I think of each one of these spots of your body as a tributary that flows to the "mouth" of the river of your inner knowing: your Oracle. And I have noticed that at a certain point, either naturally or deliberately, your Oracle will hook up (no pun intended) to your whole body's wisdom, including that of your head, heart, and gut—your thoughts, reasons, concerns, fears, emotions, and instincts.

I look forward to the day when "commune with your Oracle" is no longer considered radical but commonplace. It will signify that we women aren't routinely overlooking a powerful source of wisdom in our bodies, one that can also act as a focal point for and synthesizer of our whole body's wisdom.

Look, if after trying out all this Oracle stuff, you find that you access your inner knowing in your big toe, hallelujah. Feminine Genius is anything but formulaic. But for now, I suggest you focus on the place of intelligence that is your Oracle, because it is, in my experience, the place where women are most disconnected. And when a woman gets reconnected to her Oracle, it is the place through which she can source the most power, fulfillment, and insight. I have seen over and over that when a woman gives communing with her Oracle a real, earnest shot, she taps into an aspect of her Genius that is entirely unreachable any other way.

your Oracle is an organ of truth

DOUBTS, DELUSIONS, FEARS, AND REASONS

Let's look more closely at the other doubts that may come up as you begin to engage with your Oracle. At the very moment you part your lips to say word one to your Oracle, you might pause and think, "Wait a minute. Whose voice will I be hearing, exactly? How, exactly, can I trust what I hear? Since my Oracle is in my sexual center, isn't my Oracle only about sex? Is that really my highest guidance? I want other things for myself besides sex. How do I know I'm not going to regret following her advice? I have followed my sexual urges before, and they got me into trouble. Shouldn't I go with a safer source of guidance like my head, heart, or gut?"

When I say that your Oracle is your in-house interpreter for the Divine, you may think, "But I am not God. There are people who have studied their whole lives to understand the power of all this. Isn't it arrogant to assume I know as much as they? I have so much psychological baggage that I am not to be trusted with what I hear internally. Surely, killers and psychopaths also listen to what they hear internally, and they are in no way trustworthy. Don't we need our sages, priests, lineages, rule enforcers, and teachers to keep us on the right path?"

You may think, "Can I really know what is best for me? Can I listen to *me*? Me, who, if given an inch of chocolate cake, will eat a mile of chocolate cake? Me, who, if given the chance, would sleep with the UPS guy or sleep in until noon? Me, who, if given the opportunity to show up, prefers to hide out? Me, who is a mile-high manic one day and a raging bitch the next? Me, who is just as much primal animal as rational human?"

yes. you. listen.

These are the questions that you must grapple with in learning to trust yourself and listen to your Oracle. Is it intuition or fear? Guidance or doubt? Instinct or compulsion? Good or evil? How do you know which is driving you? How do you know that what you are hearing is not just the voice of a hang-up, addiction, or past wound? How do you know if you are talking with angels or demons? How do you know if you are maneuvering with a trustable compass or about to lose control of the wheel?

I get it. These have been my questions, too. These are the questions of nearly every woman, too—of course. Worthy concerns, all. First, you can learn to discern the different voices within you, all the while respecting and befriending them. Then, it's important to go back to focusing on your Oracle because her softer, subtler voice often requires patience in order to be heard, and her symbolic, indirect guidance often requires decryption in order to be understood.

Remember Callie, whose childhood act 1 we looked in on back in chapter 3? I caught up with her a few years after we worked together. She had answered for herself that most difficult question about her relationship, "Should I stay or should I go?" Her answer was, "Go." She spent many agonizing months looking for reasons big enough to justify her leaving. Although there were plenty of reasons for her to separate from her partner—their incompatibility in communication, sex, and whether or not to have children—Callie made her decision from a place that wasn't about reasons. She made her choice by consulting with her Oracle.

There is something unmistakable about a woman who has come home to herself—a still center, a strong backbone, and a sparkling energy. I see it all over Callie, even over our video call. When we talk, she is living with her new love, Adam.

"Looking for reasons can be ugly because you will find them," she tells me, tearing up a little. "I really had to first get in touch with my own sexual energy and see it as a kind of life-force energy. I could then be in my body and feelings (and Oracle!) in a different way than before in my life. So then, I really just kept asking myself, 'what do I want?' and from that place—before any reasons—my answer was clear. It really took something to get to know myself and what all my voices—my fear voice, my desire voice, my higher-self voice, my parent's voice—sound like." Callie's are the words of a woman who has learned how to trust her Oracle, and thereby to trust herself.

> We have been raised to fear the yes
> within ourselves, our deepest cravings.
> **AUDRE LORDE**

As the voice of your Oracle becomes stronger, and you feel more sure of it, you find it easier to trust what you hear. You hear the voice of your Oracle as distinct from the voices of delusion, fear, reason, or addiction. And, as you keep walking the path of Feminine Genius, it becomes easier to find the wisdom even *within* the voices of delusion, fear, reason, or addiction.

Discerning Your Inner Voices

As you know, you've got all kinds of voices within you that are happy to chime in given even the tiniest invitation: your five senses, your intuition, your emotions, impulses, instincts, urgings, warnings, fears, judgments, and reasons. How's a girl to hear her Oracle in that kind of cacophony, let alone trust it? Let's take a closer look at each of them, so you can begin to distinguish them for yourself, all the while confirming that each is your friend, not your foe. (Yes, even fear.) Each, when seen correctly and worked with skillfully, is a source of somatic intelligence, custom-designed for your learning and growth. As a way to begin your process of discernment, let me attend to some of the worthy concerns from the beginning of this chapter.

First, it's true that going with the guidance from your head, heart, or gut can be more of a sure thing than listening to your Oracle. Not to mention more socially acceptable. I mean, you can talk about your head, heart, or gut at any fancy dinner party without anyone asking you to leave. But, there comes a time when you want more. You want truth. You want passion, self-expression, and the confidence that only comes as you walk your Feminine Genius path. That time is now.

Second, if you get the guidance from your Oracle to have more and to have better nooky, she is likely on to something. Your Oracle is not just about sex. And yet, what woman couldn't do with reclaiming and reintegrating her sexual energy and letting it flow more powerfully? It is less a question of whether sexual urges can be trusted and more a question of whether you trust your own (and another's) *no* or *yes*. Do you trust your ability to get into and out of situations when you want more, or when you've had enough? Do you trust that this is *not* your last chance to get something finger-licking good, because you know that the Universe won't ever run out?

Last, it is good to remember that, although your Oracle makes her home in your (spicy) sexual center, she is all about the other (mild and medium) expressions of erotic energy and pleasure as well: creativity, well-being, communion, and meaning. Your Oracle's job is tending your light and fire, period.

But here is the thing. The voice of your Oracle feels *completely* different from delusion, fear, reason, or compulsion. Let me share with you some of the distinctions I have gathered with clients and participants over the years, to help you to distinguish—and befriend—each voice for yourself. Then learning to listen to your Oracle first, and all the other domineering voices later, will allow you to sift the chaff of an untruth from the wheat of your truth.

Fight, Flight, Freeze, Feed, Flock, and Fornicate

There is a part of your brain that is affectionately called the lizard brain, partly because, in terms of biology and evolution, it is the oldest part the brain, and partly because it is about all a lizard has for brain function. It is the primitive part of our human brain that we share with other animals, and is responsible for primal functions like breathing, coordination, and balance, and survival urges like defense, eating, and mating.

Your lizard brain is the part of you on hyper-vigilant alert and, when "triggered," will demand you "freak out," through fighting, fleeing, freezing, feeding, flocking—or fornicating. Fighting, fleeing, and freezing are pretty self-explanatory, but I add three more *F*s. By *feed*, I mean the instinct to put food in your body, whether consciously or compulsively. By *flock*, I mean the impulse to do what the group is doing, to keep up with the Joneses, and to not rock the boat. By *fornicate*, I mean the urge to jump in the sack with someone who is probably bad news for you. Your lizard brain is responsible for two things: making sure you don't die, and making sure you reproduce. Your lizard brain will use the six *F*s as it sees fit.

Your lizard brain doesn't always distinguish between real or imagined danger. It doesn't concern itself with the concept of time, and in many ways, it hasn't yet learned that you grew up. That you made it out alive. That you are actually quite lithe, discerning, smart, and strong. That you are no longer dependent on pleasing someone so they will feed you, love you, keep a roof over your head, or wipe your butt.

Reasoning: Judgment and Deceit

There is another part of your brain that is called your prefrontal cortex, which is the "reasoning" part of your brain. This reasoning, judging, analytical brain—the headquarters of your Masculine Genius—allows you to do and comprehend truly amazing things, like music, writing, physics, and philosophy. And yet it is this same part of your mind that also allows you to lie, whether to yourself or another, as it seems only human beings can.

As the dominant culture believes, you might also believe that the rational brain defines you as a human being and separates you from lower—and lowlier—forms of life, like lizards. Your rational brain (Masculine Genius) thinks it is the boss and tries valiantly to run the whole show, trying to do your soul's job (Feminine Genius). But really, your rational brain is working above its pay grade. As Dolano, a satsang and meditation teacher I sat with in India, puts it, "Your mind is trying to be your master when its real job is your beloved servant." Your rational brain hasn't yet had time to appreciate the power and accuracy of your Oracle. In time, it will stop trying to drive and will instead upgrade to beloved devotee of Feminine Genius.

Even Our Foolish Brains Can Be Wise

Compulsion, obsession, addiction, delusion, garden-variety fears, and the "reasonable" voice that warns you off "indulgences"—such as a lifelong passion for watercolor painting that you deny because your brain labels it as neither practical nor dignified (even though you feel deliciously alive when you paint)—come from both the lizard and rational parts of your brain. Some schools of thought instruct that these voices of fear, addiction, or analysis are parts of you that want to "keep you small," sabotage you, or inflate your sense of self to delusional proportions. The instruction is to then treat these parts of you (often called your ego) as an invading cancer—something foreign that wants the worst for you.

But this is a misguided instruction. If you subscribe to this criminalization of your voices of fear, addiction, or analysis, you then walk around assuming you have hellions within you just waiting to do you in and, who knows, perhaps just waiting to do others in as well. I believe if you look closely, you will see that there is nowhere you could go, nothing you could do, and nothing you could feel or think, where the Divine is not. Even in your judgments and fear-based thinking. Even in your ego. God is in your lizard brain and rational brain, too. You do not have a force for evil lurking in your head. Actually, you *do* have a potential force for evil lurking in your head, but only if you treat what's in your head as evil.

It is not about *having* voices of fear, addiction, or analysis. It is about how you *regard* those voices of fear, addiction, or analysis. As you learned in navigating your dark emotions, anything like fear, doubt, smallness, greed, anger, lust, blame, intolerance, hatred, or otherwise needs to be recognized, not as the enemy but as a part of you. When treated badly, these parts behave badly. Go after them like adversaries, and they will cower and fester in your dark recesses. (See, wasn't our romp through the underworld in part one worth it? You're welcome.)

Feminine Genius sways you to believe instead that every part of you is rooting for you, not against you. When each part is recognized with dignity and respect, it can transform into a wise messenger. Every cast-off part needs a promotion, not a firebombing. After all, your brain is part of your body. Every aspect of your brain and body loves you utterly. Every aspect of you has a positive intention for you, such as keeping you safe, loved, belonging, learning, growing, valued, and self-expressed. Every aspect, without exception.

However, your voices of fear, addiction, or analysis usually miss the mark in terms of what they propose you *do* in order to feel safe, loved, belonging, learning, growing, valued, and self-expressed. They often suggest actions that are at odds with the brilliance of your being, like: "Hide under the covers for the rest of your life." "Just one more martini." "I *deserve* this third pint of ice cream!" "Why yes,

I will go home with you; my husband will never find out." Or "Look and act perfect so no one finds out you are a fraud." But these voices are not the enemy. They are you. They are another form of intelligence—to be deciphered, admittedly—and hold key information for you as you learn and grow.

INTUITION, SENSATIONS, AND EMOTIONS

Then there is the intelligence of your intuitive, feeling body—a whole other set of inner voices. Listening to your Oracle requires you to become fluent with the language of your intuition, sensations, feelings, and emotions.

Intuition, my dictionary confirms for me, is defined as spiritual perception, the ability to understand something immediately and directly, without the need for conscious reasoning. I also consider intuition to be your sixth sense. Along with your five senses of sight, smell, taste, touch, and hearing, your intuition helps you receive important—and sacred—information. I have noticed, too, that intuition couples nicely with self-esteem. Meaning, the more you hold yourself in a healthy regard, the more intuitive guidance you are likely to receive, the more you are able to trust what you hear, and the more you are able to trust yourself to follow what you hear. Listening to your intuitive Oracle inherently allows you to become more comfortable with who you are.

The voices of your intuition, senses, sensations, and emotions are often quieter and softer, harder to understand than cognitive thought and strong impulses. Thoughts and reasons from your cognitive brain and lizard brain like to jump in quickly and manhandle your intuitive feelings like a Tokyo commuter in the crush of rush hour. So, after you experience your senses, sensations, emotions, and intuitions, you might be flooded with interpretations, analysis, reasons, labels, and language, which occur at more complex, abstracted levels of perception. And still, your softer, quieter, intuitive voices prefer to amble along like a Southern belle with all the time in the world.

The voices of reason or the freaked-out commands of the six *F*s—fight, flight, freeze, feed, flock, and fornicate—can easily override your intuitive perceptions. We live in a world that is so loud, overbearing, demanding, and full of reasons that it can be particularly hard for us to hear our quiet truth. And because we are culturally groomed as girls and women to follow someone else's script, it can be particularly hard for us to hear and trust our desires, impulses, and intuition in the first place. When you are "in your head" and "out of your body," you often think, reason, and judge yourself into a confused frenzy. Getting "out of your head" and "into your body" can often reconnect you with your feelings, needs, desires, clarity, and truth.

And yet, at first it may not be obvious what part of you is speaking. Intuition or reason? Oracle or lizard brain? For example, let's say you are asked to speak to several hundred people on a topic you care deeply about. You ask yourself if you should accept the invitation, and you get a response of *heck, no.* You wonder if you are hearing a trustable *no* or a knee-jerk compulsion to hide. Is it a fear voice warning you from what actually could be a very good move for you? Who has the mic, your intuitive Oracle, your frightened lizard, or your cocksure cortex? If you decline the offer, will you be moving the way fear or over-reasoning makes you move, or the way your soul asks you to move?

What these varied voices feel like, and where and how you feel them is entirely personal and will differ from woman to woman, but here are some generalities to help you discern for yourself.

- The voice of your Oracle usually feels calm but enlivening, steady and direct.

- The voice of your Oracle is often felt in your low belly, pelvis, and sometimes in your solar plexus, with feelings of expansion, opening, breath, clarity, solidity, and self-esteem.

- (As an aside, I have a hunch that oftentimes a "gut feeling" is often actually an "Oracle feeling," as your Oracle is geographically right next to your intestinal tract.)

- The voice of fear often feels wavering, vacillating, and shaky.

- The voices of compulsion and addiction are often felt in your head, neck, shoulders, chest, or upper belly, with feelings of anxiety, worry, desperation, mania, lack of control, and self-loathing.

- Your Oracle's *no* can come with feelings of clarity, solidity, and self-affirmation; while a fear-based, addiction-based, or analytical-based *no* can come with feelings of confusion, compulsion, vitriol, and self-doubt.

- Your Oracle's *yes* can come with feelings of clarity, solidity, and self-affirmation; while a fear-based, addiction-based, or analytical-based *yes* can come with feelings of confusion, compulsion, mania, and self-doubt.

I was quite intrigued when Leigh, a teacher of Vajrayana Tantric Buddhism, called the "diamond path" or "path of desire," joined my mentorship program. I was curious to see how my provocative viewpoints might overlap with her distinguished Buddhist lineage. Although she grew up in a small town in Canada, Leigh and her family are Zulu, and moved from South Africa when she was a young girl. She wanted our work together to help her *embody* many of her beloved philosophies, including embracing bodily desires as a path to enlightenment. (For so many women, embracing our bodily desires as a path to anything other than trouble is such a hot topic that I gave it its own chapter, coming up next.)

Leigh had spent countless hours on her beloved meditation cushion, studying detailed sketches of how energy moves in the body—a map of enlightenment. Yet, while any map is useful, a map simply isn't the journey. Leigh's philosophies had remained ideas in her mind, and she used the laboratory of our program together to live and breathe the philosophies.

As she put it, "Learning from high esoteric scriptures *points* the way, but it won't get you there. You have to experience it viscerally and subjectively through your body. Whereas the philosophies I learned *described* a flower, in our program together you said, 'go *experience* the flower—the red, the softness, the smell—and later add the label of *flower.*'" Leigh put her sensuous, desirous, wildly feeling female body *first*, and then gave her mind the job of processing it all afterward.

Beatific, Leigh smiled at me through my computer screen and concluded, "There was no need to kick out anything that I learned from my lineage, but I did need to flip the order. So, first body, then mind. Because I'm going to become enlightened through *my body*, through my embodied visceral experience." Leigh asked her reasoning mind to help keep her on her path, but she asked her body to lead the way.

> Your body is precious.
> It is your vehicle for awakening.
> **BUDDHA**

Recovering your ability to simply know what you know—as was likely commonplace at some point in your girlhood—is a natural byproduct of befriending and deciphering all parts of yourself. Friend, Feminine Genius isn't interested in you *transcending* your body. Feminine Genius needs you *in* your body so she can speak with you, through your Oracle.

And you, dear one, can trust your Oracle to guide you home.

14

Your Very Own Pandora's Box
Unearthing Your Desires

Re-kindling desire is basically the transition from
numb to alive, ordinary to extraordinary, profane to
sacred, productive to playful, separate to connected.
ESTHER PEREL

You want a compass? An inner guidance system by which to navigate your crazy, splendid life? You've got one, sister. It's your Oracle.

What calls you out on the open road with your Oracle at the wheel, what directs you to the place where *X* marks the spot, what compels you to kneel down and start digging—are your desires. The Pandora's box that you bring up from where it has been buried—contains your desires.

Your desires are what you want, what you strongly long for. Your desires, heroine, are the call to adventure. Your desires are your cool soul's instructions mixed with your body's lust for life, tugging at you, whispering to you, and pulling you along your path. Yet, what woman among us doesn't have a fraught relationship with her desires?

Your desires, alas, are generally neither simple nor straightforward. Each desire is a unique fusion of the inner voices you just distinguished in the last chapter. It's like this: find yourself a nice big treasure chest and into it pour some sensations and a few emotions; a big splash of intuition; a couple instincts, impulses, and urges; and a double dose of longing. Mix vigorously, and then garnish with a doubt and a delusion or two, and voilà! You've got yourself one delicious Pandora's box of desires.

Pandora, if you don't know her, is a much-maligned, mythical female, famous for lifting the lid of the very box she was told not to, led by her desire to understand the mystery of what lay within. She certainly isn't the first (or only) woman to be condemned for her disobedience, shamed for her longings, and blamed for letting loose all manner of torments and troubles into the world.

But not everyone interprets Pandora's myth as a cautionary tale of how evil came to the world—through a woman. One understanding of the name *Pandora* is "she who sends up gifts." In an alternate interpretation of her story, Pandora embodies the sexy fertility of the earth and its capacity to "send up gifts" such as seeds and fruits and pearls and other treasures for the benefit of all humankind.

And yet, you may be wary about listening to your Oracle, lifting the lid of your desires, and letting your longing loose in the world. Aren't your desires the very things that limit your awareness, dumb down your human potential, lead you astray, and propel you compulsively toward pleasure one moment and away from pain the next? Not necessarily. As my friend and author Jena la Flamme says, "Desire is not the same thing as compulsion, addiction, or unconscious consumption, though many people mistakenly confuse them."

As a human and as a woman, your desires can be some of the most exalted parts of you, not some of the least. Your desires are the longings of the Universe, longing to be lived *through* you and *as* you. Your Oracle's specialty is alerting you to your desires. As the thirteenth-century Persian mystic poet Rumi says, "Your longing for the Divine *is* divine." Letting your Oracle alert you to your desires and steer you in their direction will keep you forever walking on the path of Feminine Genius.

Each desire is a complex amalgam of lead and gold, of delusion and vision, of the sensual and the spiritual, of trouble and treasure. A desire can be just as easily G-rated as X-rated. It can be mild, medium, or spicy. A desire can be simple or multidimensional, Technicolor, and elaborate. A desire can be a prescient nudge, a creative impulse, a simple truth, or an inspired vision. A desire can be a tangible, actionable, obtainable thing or experience, directing you to "visit the pyramids in Egypt," "take a week off," "get a massage every week," or "learn how to have multiple, full-body orgasms."

Nevertheless, desires need to be honed. Without opening the lid on your Pandora's box and examining the contents, you just don't really know what kinds of jewels—and what kinds of challenges—lie inside. And that's part of the point. Sorting through your desire's contradictions to find the jewels of truth inside is as much the point as is fulfilling any desire. Getting what you want is not nearly as important as what you must learn—and who you must become—as you try to get it.

HONING YOUR DESIRES

One hot August afternoon over a decade ago, I sat on the steps of a Manhattan brownstone with my friend and mentor Regena Thomashauer (aka Mama Gena) while she savored a cigarette. For some reason, she got me talking about my early twenties, a time I refer to as my "early midlife crisis" period. I had left my fancy college dance program to "find myself" by living on my own in a strange city far from home, newly of legal drinking age.

I told Regena about a habit I developed where I would stalk unsuspecting yet handsome young men in dive bars as a valiant attempt to meet my soul mate. At the time, I didn't really see it as a problem because I was such an easygoing, charming, and well-intentioned stalker. However, each guy, without exception, sometime between date one and date two, would literally say out loud to my face, "I am not your soul mate." But I would sleep with him again once or thrice just to be sure. "My desires were all messed up. I just didn't have good inner wisdom at that time in my life," I told Regena.

"Oh no, darling," she told me. "Your desires were working just fine. You were *developing* your inner wisdom."

Oh, I realized. *I'm not deficient in inner wisdom. It can be developed.* I felt a little less troubled and a little more wise. Too stunned to say much else, I said, "Huh. Wow. Well, thank you!"

"You're welcome. But next time, try, 'thank you, it's true.'" Regena winked at me. "Might as well admit you're pretty great, mess and all."

As it turns out—and what I took from my conversation with my mentor—although your desires are natural and wise, they aren't necessarily good to go right out of the mouth of your Oracle. Although your desires are transmissions from Feminine Genius herself, they also come through your unique, wounded, wonderful psyche and body. The woman who can hear the voice of her soul speak to her through her Oracle is the same woman who learned early on that she should not speak until spoken to, that a lady closes her legs when she sits, that she is not as smart as her brother, that she should look pretty so she doesn't end up a poor spinster, that boys are only after one thing, that everything that feels good is bad, and that it is all up to her so she has to do it all herself.

As it turns out, you aren't meant to simply fulfill an unexamined desire, but instead to chip away at each surface-level desire to reveal the deep desire inside. However much a desire might be a holy messenger, it still needs to be honed. This honing process—opening the lid of the box, peering inside, sorting rock from gem, burning away lead to lay bare veins of gold—requires ever-expanding self-awareness and discernment.

You know you are in the honing process when you make a mess, fall on your face, and then ask yourself, "What would I do better next time? If I look back with what I know now, what wisdom was at play that I couldn't see then? From that experience, what do I want to toss and what do I want to keep?"

My desire as a twenty-something to find a soul mate wasn't inherently flawed. I had to try a few (or twenty) one-night stands to hone my desires and to turn up the volume on my inner wisdom. I would love to save you a few unwanted one-night stands and a few unnecessary empty tequila bottles; however, learning to trust your Oracle and hone your desires through the process of trial and error is as it is designed to be.

Surface Desire versus Deep Desire

In a moment, I'll lead you through an exercise that is designed to help you excavate the deep desire inside a surface desire. A surface desire is *still* a desire, and it can feel urgent, such as wanting to eat an entire chocolate cake, quit your job, or hop in the sack with the UPS guy. But ultimately, your surface desire might not be fulfilling. And it might leave you with a bellyache, a headache, or a long spell of regret.

To use the UPS guy as an example, the *surface* aspect of your desire might be for sex with that hot guy toting your packages, but your *deeper* desire might be for something like: life-force running through your body; spontaneity; being able to say *yes* to an opportunity that literally comes knocking on your door; spiritual union; feeling desirable and attractive; or changing the sexual agreements in your marriage to include having intimacy and sex with others.

If you just go with the surface desire and hop in bed with the UPS guy, you could miss the deeper wisdom and reasons embedded within your desire, and you could do something that violates your personal ethics. However, once you learn to distinguish your surface from deep desires, you can start to figure out ways to get your deep desires met without necessarily trampling on your boundaries and values.

DESIRE PRACTICE   **SORTING SURFACE FROM DEEP DESIRES**

Don't be scared by the length of this practice. The more you do it, the more natural and effortless it will become, so what used to be a series of in-depth contemplations will eventually be just a few moments of self-inquiry.

1 Pick one of your desires. A desire is an experience, understanding, or thing that you want, that you long for, that enlivens you, that calls to you. If you are having trouble accessing what you want, you can check in with the *yes* feelings in your body. Or, you can ask your Oracle, "What do I desire?" If it is helpful, you can remind yourself

it is safe to know your desires, and you can thank yourself
for the courage to share your desires.

2　With curiosity rather than judgment, ask yourself (or your
Oracle) some or all of the following questions and write
(or record) the answers you receive:
  • When this desire is met, what will I *feel* (emotions,
    impulses, and sensations)?
  • When this desire is met, what will I *know about
    myself* (beliefs, abilities, capabilities, sense of self,
    frames of mind)?
  • What feels *most important* about meeting this desire?
  • Assuming there is a rebellious, disgruntled teenager
    in me, what might that part of me be acting out
    against, moving away from, proving or disproving,
    reclaiming or avoiding by having this desire?
  • Assuming there is a vulnerable, unsafe-feeling,
    small child in me, what might that part of me be
    defending, protecting, numbing to, attempting to
    fix, trying to save, or simply hoping for by having
    this desire?
  • How might this desire *positively* impact me/my
    partner/my family/my community (in ways perhaps
    not easily seen at first glance)?
  • How might this desire *negatively* impact me/my
    partner/my family/my community (in ways perhaps
    not easily seen at first glance)?

3　Find a "baby step"—a small chunk of this desire—to
experiment with. Ask yourself (or your Oracle) the
following questions as a guide. You can also enlist help
from a friend or partner, if you want.
  • Are there easier, simpler, more effective ways that will
    have less impact on me/my partner/my family/my
    community to get some or all of this desire met?

- What is the smallest chunk of this desire that I could experiment with and use as research to get more information?

4 *After* you experiment with your "baby step," make sure to self-reflect on these questions:
- What worked?
- What didn't work?
- What would I like to repeat, and what would I like to *not* repeat?
- What about the experiment am I most grateful for?
- What do I want my next step to be?

FOLLOWING YOUR DESIRES

Following your desires is one of the keys to living a Feminine Genius life and becoming the woman you long to be. But it's also no joke. When she calls, or you call her in, there is just as likely to be a joy storm as a shit storm.

I experienced this firsthand with my friend Sera, an author and recovering Harvard-trained comparative religions scholar. One evening, Sera was taking a break from writing to let other humans visit, and I was the lucky human. Generally, Sera preferred to hang out with the Divine Feminine (who can blame her?), her trash-talking parrot, Anaya, and her tiny Chihuahua, Lalla, who is named after the often-naked Sufi mystic poetess and who has a compulsive and mostly endearing licking habit. The dog licked, I mean. About the naked poetess, I couldn't say.

While we ate take-out Burmese food, Sera showed me a newspaper article from the *New York Times* in which she was featured, along with two of her friends, as three women to watch as rising stars in the world of fresh voices for young women's spirituality. She had a dazzling list of opportunities knocking at her door and promising projects she was in the middle of—even Oprah was expressing interest. But her inner guidance had said no, to all of them. So, she had shakily said no, as well. She explained to me that the guidance she was listening to was the voice of her soul—or as I call it, Feminine Genius, which, as you know by now, often has other plans for you than what you have planned.

At the time, with a plate of spicy noodles on my lap and a tiny dog licking my arm, I thought that Sera should hang up on her soul and get back on the line with Oprah. But over the years, I started to feel the power, the essence, the energy, the truth, and the intelligence of what it was that Sera was listening to and acting on. I started to glimpse what is more precious than the gold stars of achievement, and I started to understand why any of us might pick tuning in to our Feminine Genius over tuning in to Oprah.

(As an aside, I freakin' love Oprah Winfrey. A woman who embodies self-esteem and who has created an empire while modeling how to responsibly wield wealth and power? Who has dedicated her life to empowering others to live truer and more meaningful lives? More, please. However, neither she nor whatever she endorses is a substitute for your own inner guidance.)

Steering your life by your desires is not about guaranteeing one particular outcome or another. It's about the quiet fulfillment that comes from a path well walked and the radical sovereignty that comes from coming home to yourself.

Oh, the places you and your desires will go! The world you will remake as you walk! The life you will reclaim as you go! Dear One, listen.

Through your desires
Feminine Genius whispers to you

LIFE IN THE FIELD

Remember how Feminine Genius likes to make her home more in quantum reality than in Newtonian reality (back in chapter 4)? Let me introduce to you the quantum phenomenon of a "field," an invisible, nonmaterial, organizing, intelligent energy. You might also be familiar with it from the work of Carl Jung, the Swiss psychoanalyst who brought us the idea of archetypes and the collective unconscious. The quantum field is the shared mind, the collective memory, or the collective soul.

Scientific experimentation with quantum fields begins to explain things such as dream sharing, telepathy, premonition, precognition, telekinesis, limb regeneration, remote viewing, garden-variety intu-ition, and the phenomenon wherein groups of the same species of animals who are separated by great geographical distances learn to do the same new skill at generally the same time, or learn a skill that pre-vious generations knew how to do, but was forgotten for long spans of time. The idea of the quantum field helps to explain how specific habits and beliefs are passed down through the "emotional DNA" of human family systems, and then expressed by family members who, often, have never met.

Rupert Sheldrake, a biologist and researcher of quantum fields, says;

> Magnetic fields extend beyond the surfaces of magnets;
> the Earth's gravitational field extends far beyond the
> surface of the Earth, keeping the moon in its orbit; and
> the fields of a cell phone stretch out far beyond the
> phone itself. Likewise the fields of our minds extend far
> beyond our brains [and bodies]. Fields . . . do most of
> the things that souls were believed to do.[1]

The tugs and pulls of the Universe that quantum researchers refer to as a field, I call your soul. Your soul, our soul—same thing. As writer Lynn McTaggart puts it, a field is like a phone network and all parts are always on the line. Your desires are the voice of the collective soul calling out to be lived through you and as you. And your Oracle picks up the call.

As women tapping into our desires and tapping into Feminine Genius, we are using the same forces that are at work in a quantum field. As we feel and intuit and hone our desires, we are in conversation with a larger, soul-based field that extends beyond our human bodies into the collective, shared consciousness. Our desires are an interface between an extrasensory field and our sensory-based world, between our soul and our workaday existence, between our Feminine Genius and our female bodies, between the other world and this one.

Our desires are also the blueprints for futures yet to be. In a quantum reality, where time and space are simply suggestions, it is as Rupert Sheldrake suggests: "Each individual inherits a collective memory from past members of the species, and also contributes to the collective memory, affecting other members of the species in the future."[2] Our desires will change who we, individually and collectively, will become. Our desires will change who we, individually and collectively, remember ourselves to be.

> Desires are memories of the future.
> **NISHA MOODLEY**

When you excavate a deep desire and then let that truth loose into the world, you not only affect yourself and your own destiny, but you also affect humankind backward and forward in time, now and in the future. You create waves that will be felt by women and men you have never seen or met, on the opposite side of the world or in an inaccessible culture. Your desires come from the other world—the world of soul, spirit, mystery, creative energy, and divine intelligence. When you follow your desires, and hone them as you go, they will lead you and me right into a new world-to-be that is richer, brighter, more aligned with truth and beauty than the one you and I are in right now. What you *feel*, what you *know*, and what you *desire*, will change the world.

Feminine Genius—the feminine flavor of God, the intelligent energy of our collective soul—loves to get your attention through your desires. A woman in this kind of intimate, ongoing conversation with the collective soul is a living embodiment of Feminine Genius. Your desires have something brilliant to tell you, if you would only unearth the treasure box and listen in. And your Oracle makes a lovely gateway for your desires to make their way into this world.

> You suppose you are the trouble, but you are the cure.
> **RUMI**

15

Calling Your Oracle
All Roads Lead You Home

What's in a name? That which we call a rose
By any other name would smell as sweet.
WILLIAM SHAKESPEARE, *Romeo and Juliet*

Your Oracle is about knowing. Knowing your desires, knowing your truth, knowing your next move, and knowing yourself as divine, and knowing how to get yourself back on track if you wobble and veer off.

Your inner knowing knows.

And yet, how I hear my inner knowing will be very different from how you hear yours. To hear your inner knowing, you may have to prick up your "soul ears"—your metaphysical organs of perception with which you listen to and sense your *internal* world as well as the *other* world (the worlds of your desires and our collective soul) rather than the *external* world. I want to pass along some useful tools and practices so that you can learn your Oracle's personal, sophisticated voice, engage her in a more personal, sophisticated dialogue, and perhaps call her by a more personal, sophisticated name. And so that should she fall silent, you can call her back to life.

Oracles are translators of the collective soul. And thus, with this illustrious job description, they are sometimes literal, but more often symbolic. As Carolyn Myss, a medical intuitive and author says:

> Past the language of logic, past the language of language
> comes the language of symbols. And it is in the language
> of symbols that you understand, decode, or discern what
> heaven is saying to you, or what your dream world is
> saying to you. It is through the language of symbols that
> you reach the interior of your soul.[1]

Oracles love to mix metaphors, images, poetry, thoughts, feelings, longings, instincts, grunts, nudges, depth, and levity, all adding up to a deep sense of inner knowing. Stay tuned for practices to help you decrypt your Oracle's particular language of symbols.

RE-NAMING YOUR ORACLE

Look, I know this is unusual and radical. Here I am calling your nethers your *Oracle*. Here I am, asking you to do a call and response with your lady parts. And here I am, taking yet another step further by inviting you (in the forthcoming Calling Your Oracle practice) to personalize your Oracle's name. Although it may at first seem frivolous, what you call your body parts is actually meaningful. As you will see in just a moment, it will transport you to the land of the symbolic.

I mean, what did your lady parts, your genitals, your female reproductive organs, get called when you were growing up? By what name did you learn to call these parts of yourself? When I ask this of my groups, I get a long, colorful list. Cutesy names like coochie or hoohah; vague and mysterious names like *down there*; sassy names like va-jay-jay or honey pot; confusing names like beaver or muffin; anatomically correct names like vulva or vagina; every once in a while I hear something complimentary like yoni or goddess.

In this crazy world, our lady parts get derogatory names like cunt, pussy, gash, and hole—and those are the ones at the polite end of the spectrum. Even the term *vagina*, however accurate, means "sheath," the receptacle into which one puts a sword. Often, women report that their genitals never even got a name or a term at all. Just silence. Nothing at all. It is hard to call upon something you don't have a name for, in a place you never thought to look.

As Eve Ensler writes in *The Vagina Monologues*, "What we don't say we don't see, acknowledge, or remember. What we don't say becomes a secret, and secrets often create shame and fear and myths."[2] Naming is needed. Re-naming is needed. A re-naming that takes your divinity and unique soul's path into account is needed. You don't *have to* listen in, ask, and name your Oracle something unique and special. There is no one right way to do this. Your Oracle, by whatever name you call her, is crucial to feeling turned *on*, rather than switched *off*.

call her what you will
but for the love of the Goddess, call her.

After doing the practice that follows, Melissa, a participant in one of my digital courses reported:

> Her name is Nahla/Nala. Some meanings: drink of water (Arabic); successful (some African languages); stem or hollow reed (Sanskrit); "I eat" (Swahili). When I asked her what she wants, she said to engage in daily serpentine belly dance and circular yogic practice. So far, this practice has evoked intense joy, feelings of liberation, and the release of repressed anger and choking sobs. This is earth-shattering progress that feels very chaotic (but safe). Nala also wants to sing, and play in the desert, and celebrate her femininity. I'm off to quite a start.

One of my mentees, Deva, who is an energy healer and quite comfortable in the realms of the mystical, didn't know what to make of the name she heard at first. "I keep hearing *Angela*, spoken with the accent and big hair of a Jersey girl," she said. When she researched the name Angela, she came up with "messenger of God, the feminine form of 'angel,' she who knows, and friendly and easy to get along with." Deva appreciated the mix of gravitas, humor, and hairspray.

Katrine, from another of my mentorship programs, heard *Rose*. At first, she was disappointed because to her, roses were boring and ordinary. After researching a bit, Katrine found that the rose is one of the most beautiful and significant symbols, sharing spiritual resonance with the Holy Grail—as in a receptive vessel of the soul, receiving the in-pouring of divine influence.

Katrine also found that the rose is essentially the Western equivalent of the Eastern lotus, as a symbol of the unfolding of higher consciousness. Members of the Sisterhood of the Rose include incarnations of the Divine Feminine, such as Isis in Egypt, Kwan-Yin in Asia, and the Black Madonna (also known as Saint Mary Magdalene) in Europe.

Other participants have reported hearing names as personal and sophisticated as Sophia, Sunshine, Kitty, Blue, Elle, Meow, Heartguts, Jane, Rosa Mexicana, Foxy Roxy, Baby, Belle, Heather, Eden, and the sound of the yogic chant *om*.

Oh, Oracles: often witty, but always profound.

So have fun trying out this simple practice of naming or re-naming your Oracle. Most importantly, it will help you to listen to your Oracle, to deepen the dialogue between you, and to get you familiar with the personal and sophisticated ways your Oracle speaks to you. So that when you want to know your truth, your next move, and yourself as Divine, eventually your question will not be, "What would Oprah do?" or "What would Jesus do?" It will become, "What would my Oracle do?"

ORACLE PRACTICE #3   CALLING YOUR ORACLE

1   Sit or stand comfortably and place your hands on your low belly, your Oracle.

2   Take a few circular waterfall breaths, imagining each in-breath as a cool breeze or a warm caress, waking

up, turning on, nourishing, soothing, or enlivening
your Oracle. Imagine each out-breath shooting out
the top of your head and cascading out in front of
you like a waterfall.

3 Direct your awareness to your body, under your
hands, and ask your Oracle the following questions
and listen for her answers.
- Ask, "What do you desire?" Listen for her answer.
- Ask, "What is important for me to know?" Listen
  for her answer.
- Ask, "What do you want to be called?" Listen for
  her answer.

4 As you are listening for her answers, use your "soul
ears" to listen/feel/sense/observe internally, the
way you would if a doctor asked you to explain the
feeling and location of a particular pain in your
abdomen without pointing to it.
- Her answers might come in the form of
  sensations, impulses, and emotions (like your *yes*
  and *no*).
- Her answers might come in the form of words
  and straightforward, straight-talking sentences.
- Her answers might come in the form of
  poetry fragments, images, grunts, symbols,
  metaphors, and nudges, perhaps requiring your
  interpretation, like dreams.

5 When you get her answer to the question, "What do
you want to be called?" go do a little research. Even
a quick online search will do. Even if you already
know what the word or name means, you may be
astounded by what else you find and its significance
for you.

There is no right way for your Oracle's answers to come, but they will come

What if You Hear Nothing?

Now, you might be wondering what to do if your Oracle's answers *don't* come. What if you ask and are met with silence? What should you do if you are trying all the questions from the previous practice and getting zip, nada, nothing? What if you are getting some kind of response you don't know how to interpret?

Your Oracle might currently be on mute, and you simply haven't yet found where you left the remote control. But your Oracle is not broken. Your Oracle works, and works well. Every single woman on the planet has her own personal, highly functioning Oracle, if only she'd dust her off and give her a whirl. Even if you don't have all your lady parts or disowned your femininity a long time ago, you absolutely have an Oracle waiting to give you a hearty, sassy earful.

Following is a practice to help your Oracle speak up. It is inspired by the simple and profound idea I first encountered in Neale Donald Walsch's book *Conversations with God*. If the practice in Walsch's book is new to you, it is essentially a two-way journaling session with you and God, inspiring this call and response with your Oracle. You can do it using the written word (pen and paper or otherwise) or spoken word (recording device), whichever suits you.

This exercise, Conversations with Your Oracle, is especially good for cryptic and silent Oracles. It is simple: write out (or speak out) a question to your Oracle, and write out (or speak out) what you hear, even if what you hear isn't an obvious answer but more of a silence, a symbol, a sensation, an emotion, an image, a sound, a line from a poem, an impulse, and so forth.

Keep going: ask, listen; ask, listen; ask, listen. Keep asking your questions (perhaps the ones listed in the Calling Your Oracle practice) and listening for her answers. For example:

ME   Hi, Oracle. Why can't I hear you?
ORACLE *silence. (static.)*

ME   I am curious about the static I hear. What's that about?
ORACLE *i am feeling upset. (harrumph.)*

ME   Oh, wow. Why?
ORACLE *i have been feeling ignored for a long time.*

ME   That's true. I'm sorry.
ORACLE *silence. (simmering water. steam.)*

ME   Will you accept my apology?
ORACLE *oh, of course. always.*
(bubbles. shooting stars.)
i am glad you called me up.

ME   Me, too! So, now that I can hear you, what's important for me to know right now?
ORACLE *(girl child on a swing, hair flying in the breeze.)*

ME   Um, meaning I should swing more? Play more?
ORACLE *sort of, yeah, honey cakes. i — we — are feeling pretty dull. we need a shot of life energy.*

ME   This may sound dumb, but why is that important?
ORACLE *so i can help you get to where you want to go.*

ME   Oh. Yep, makes sense. And, you, is there something you would like to be called?
ORACLE *Thanks for asking, why yes there is: Alma.*

Alma is the name I heard when I first asked. Never really thought much about the name Alma before that moment. When I looked it up in the dictionary, I found that *alma* means "soul" in Spanish, "young woman" in Hebrew, "wild apple" in Hungarian, "all good" in Celtic and Irish, "loving" in Swedish, and "jump" in Greek. In English, *alma mater* refers to a place of higher education.

Well then. Wow, Oracle, now we are talking.

Now it's your turn.

ORACLE PRACTICE #4   CONVERSATIONS WITH YOUR ORACLE

This practice is helpful for loosening up cryptic and quiet Oracles. When you're writing, I suggest you use one color to indicate your questions and another color for your Oracle's answers.

1   Connect with your Oracle (perhaps by doing the Oracle Meditation practice you learned in chapter 12). Then ask her, "Why can't I hear you? What put you on mute?"

2   Listen until you hear an answer, even if the answer is silence, or it's confusing to you. Write/speak whatever you hear.

3   In call-and-response fashion, continue to ask questions that come up in response to her answers. Write/speak whatever you hear.

welcome home, Oracle

CONSULTING YOUR ORACLE AS A WAY OF LIFE

I highly recommend consulting your Oracle as a way of life. This means that when your Oracle points you in a direction, experiment with taking your Oracle's lead, even if it feels like sailing in the pitch dark out in the open ocean. Here's a little anecdote to guide us, inspired by my friend Sera: You look through your telescope and see an island off to your left and head to it. You ask, "Hey Oracle, whatcha think? Starboard direction! Looks like a great island! Head there for the night?"

Your Oracle (strangely) says, *No.*

It looks like a perfectly good island to you. Sad and disheartened, you gird your loins to sail on through the night, tired, hungry, and wet.

But, here's what: It is as though your Oracle is perched on the mast, thirty feet in the air, and can see from her vantage point that the island has no potable water and is home to swarms of malaria-carrying mosquitoes.

And, here's what: It is as though your Oracle has come down from the mast and sunk her periscope into the waters to take another look at the island. Although you could never see it from your position on the boat, she can see the massive rocks, only five feet below the water, that would without hesitation rip through the hull of your boat and sink you.

Your Oracle steers by the light of the moon. Your Oracle has night vision and can see in the dark. Your Oracle always has your back. Your Oracle is on "team you." Your Oracle's guidance will at times be great news, sweet as honey. At other times, it will burn away all that no longer serves you, and all that is no longer you. Tirelessly, she will make sure you are walking your Feminine Genius path, no matter what you need to learn or how you need to grow as you go.

all roads lead to your Oracle.
all roads lead you Home.

16

Your Body Is The Temple (and Other Heresies)

Another Cheat Sheet

You are the secret the universe is telling.

GOPALA AIYAR SUNDARAMOORTHY

The word *heresy* comes from the Greek word *hairesis*, which means "views strongly opposed to any generally accepted ideas."[1] In times other than these, I might have been drawn and quartered, flayed, or burned at the stake for the scandalous views I've shared on these pages, particularly here in part three. It's enough to drive a goddess underground. But guess what? It is springtime for wayward goddesses. And besides, a heretic was long ago simply known as *one who is able to choose*. I may indeed be a heretic, but from the relative safety of this century, let's review our choices, shall we?

You Can Speak Directly with God   Countless popes are turning over in their graves. Many a page of *O* magazine will be left unturned.

Whatever it is you have simply forgotten, you can remember. No intermediary needed. You can know yourself. Directly, keenly, authoritatively. In fact, who could truly know, but you?

Erotic Energy Is Creative Energy   Your passion and power come through integrating and owning your sensual energy, rather than by denouncing or cloistering it.

Rather than separating you from the Divine, your erotic energy is a force for divine union. Rather than leading you to ruin, Eros will lead you into the life you are aching to live.

Often, you find your truth in the least likely places.

The Godhead Isn't in Your Head   Your body is not an impediment to divinity; your body *is* divine. You can get into real-deal communion with the eternal, not by transcending your body but *through* your body, your corporeal, workaday, human body.

No need to vanquish, conquer, or control your body. No need to slay your ego before meeting the Holy One. No altar needed at which to pray for insight and inspiration.

Your body *is* the altar—and the temple.

A Rose by Any Other Name Would Smell as Sweet   The reasons, opinions, rules, and judgments of your brain are great sources of guidance. As are the compassionate, empathic urgings of your heart. As are the powerful, compelling instincts of your gut. Friends, all.

But to get to the intuitive murmurings of the soul in your belly, you must have the discipline to bring your awareness further down, into your Oracle, to hear the voices that are quieter and subtler, but connected directly to cosmic intelligence.

And it turns out, instead of a silent and shameful *down there*, you've got a sacred vessel. Thanks to your lady parts.

Guidance Comes in the Form of Your Longings   You can know your deepest truth by befriending your body's sensations, emotions, impulses, instincts, intuitions, passions, aches, and desires.

For everything you dearly want, there is someone wishing and waiting for it to be born. Your deepest desires are sent to you from a world-to-be that only you can see. Honed, your desires become precious pieces of your inner wisdom.

When Feminine Genius knocks you up, it is your sacred responsibility to grow those desire-babies into sturdy powerhouses, and then send them galloping off into the world.

Guidance Is Best Heard While Turned On   Meditative, devotional, and prayer practices that are seated, still, contemplative, serious, and thought based—are so last century.

Your enjoyment, your pleasure, your aliveness, as felt by your feeling, changing, cycling, moving woman's body, are the preferred mediums for our collective soul to have a word with you.

Cultivating your light and tending to your fire will let you hear the quiet, wise voice of your truth, and will give you the courage and confidence to follow what you hear. Nothing like a whole fourth and final section to explore this one. Will you come along with me now?

remember:

The Divine is having a human
experience through you
There is nowhere you could go
and nothing you could do
To fall from the embrace of the Beloved
you are already holy
you are already home
you are the One we are waiting for
let's go

Part Four

Cultivating Your Light

17

What You Appreciate, Appreciates
Creating a Field of Light

Out beyond wrongdoing and rightdoing is a field.
I'll meet you there.
RUMI

Welcome, woman.

You crawled through the underworld and got re-birthed, re-membered, re-educated, re-ignited, re-named, and re-united. You got yourself your own private Oracle, your always-on audience with your soul. You noticed that the voice of your truth can become bashful and soft-spoken in contrast to life's noise. You know how to listen to and learn from your desires.

Like a light bulb, you function best when you are turned on. Your light is life-force energy, as seen and felt through your body. Your light is Eros, as channeled and expressed in your quotidian life. Your light is your power. It is what powers life itself and what powers you. Your light is the fuel within you and also what radiates from you. It is what blesses life and also what blesses you. Your light is the same as divine light.

Cultivating your light means that you wake up, again and again, to the awe of being alive and at home in your body. Not someday when you are perfect, but right now, in your humble life and your quirky body just as they are. I want for you to ally yourself with your light and live there, much of the time, even as your darkness ebbs and flows within you, and even if you have felt alienated from your body, sexuality, and inner knowing until now. You can, Feminine Genius, live brilliantly ever after.

But your light requires care and tending. Your light can easily flicker when you overuse your Masculine Genius—or when you follow a script, forget how to navigate your dark, become comfortably numb, modify who you are in order to fit in, overlook that who you are is holy, and believe for too long that you are wrong, broken, or crazy. Your inner wisdom, moxie, and vibrancy all need specific conditions in which to shine. This section is all about going *up* into the light parts of the death/rebirth cycle. Because, dear one, it really takes something to tend your radiance and to know how to turn it back up when it dims.

A great by-product of walking the path of Feminine Genius and allying yourself with your light is that you will have fewer crappy experiences and more wonderful ones. Life gets better and brighter. However, becoming masterful at cultivating your light does not mean you become inoculated against difficulty. You will still experience disappointment and loss. Things will, from time to time, not go your way. You will descend again into the dark part of the death/ rebirth cycle.

None of this means that you are doing light cultivation wrong, are a bad human, or have failed Feminine Genius school. It simply means you are having a life. As you know, your life is *supposed* to go up and down. To keep walking your Feminine Genius path, you need to know how to navigate the dark times when they come, and cultivate the light times so they come more and more often.

So, in this crazy world that tends to cut off your power in the blink of a to-do list, this whole section will offer you ways to keep your power flowing. I have for you some radical ways of being, muscle-strengthening practices, and chop-honing exercises to help you enjoy yourself, come vibrantly alive, get great at receiving, express your desires, and use the power of sisterhood to keep your flame turned on. Daily, weekly, all your life long.

Let's start with creating a field of light.

THE POWER OF YOUR AWARENESS

As I see it, the only two things in life you truly have any control over are the *quality* of your awareness, and *to what* you direct your awareness. On what will you focus? Will you treasure it or trash it? Will you see it for what it is, or only for what it is not? At first glance, this may seem overly simple or obtuse, but it is actually a key to wielding your power and enjoying your life.

I first learned about the power of awareness in a strange and bass-ackward way, almost a decade ago. My partner, Nathan, and I were in a session with a well-known relationship coach, Kevin. Kevin asked me to explain my side of a communication issue between Nathan and me, but when I opened my mouth, I was literally unable to speak. I was struck mute. Instead, I squirmed, as though I were sitting on pins and needles. I felt dumb and inadequate. Tears jabbed my eyeballs. After many long minutes of this, Nathan stopped the session, took me by the elbow, and led me out to the car.

Nathan and I talked, trying to figure out what in the world had happened. How had I, a naturally articulate and forthcoming person, become unable to speak up? Slowly, we realized that the way Kevin had been listening to me, and the energy he had been broadcasting, had been shutting me down. "I got the sense that he really didn't like what you were saying. I could feel his contempt of you. And then, you stopped being able to speak," Nathan said.

Hearing my partner's insight, I calmed down and began to brush off my discomfort. *Then* I became fascinated by the power of my energetic exchange with Kevin. How he had *listened to* and *looked at* me had, directly and powerfully, affected how I spoke and how I felt about myself. Was I super-sensitive, an anomaly, or was I onto something about the ability we have to influence others, in both dark and light ways?

CREATING A FIELD OF APPRECIATION

For the next many years, I tried this out in my live retreats and programs, to the same effect every time. I would divide the group of women into pairs and have half of them leave the room to get ready to share what they were most excited to get out of the program. I gave the women present in the room their instructions: when their partners came back, they weren't to *say* anything, just *listen* to what their partner shared. They were to be deliberate about listening in a way that was generous, appreciative, and welcoming. They were to direct their awareness to the beauty and wisdom they found in their partner's face, body, and words; and they were to broadcast interest, enjoyment, and excitement.

So far, so good. But then, half way through, I would clear my throat, their signal to switch the quality of their listening and seeing. They were to continue to listen to their partner, but in a way that was harsh, judgmental, and critical. Again, without saying anything, they were to direct their awareness to the flaws they could find in their partner's face, body, and words; and they were to broadcast boredom, displeasure, and contempt.

After I gave these instructions, they looked at me as though I must be kidding. But taking it on faith that my request to do something they found repugnant might help them embody their Feminine Genius, they agreed to try it. We brought their partners back into the room. At the end of the exercise, we heard first from the partners who were speaking, the ones being listened to. Nearly universally, the speakers started out animated, inspired, and articulate. Their words flew out of them, even those usually shy, and they reported enjoying what they were sharing, and were feeling good about themselves. A few of their partners noted that they looked radiant and lovely as they spoke.

The speakers shared that then something shifted, and they sort of lost their trains of thought. "Yes," others piped in. "Somehow I lost my steam or felt like what I was saying wasn't that important." "I noticed my voice got quieter, and I wondered if I was boring my partner," a few said. When I revealed what was going on, they were surprised and awed, as I was after my disturbing coaching session with Kevin many years back. Even after we reversed roles, and everyone knew what was going on, the results were pretty much the same.

Your awareness—the way you listen to and regard another—is a *field* of energy that transmits and broadcasts, like a radio signal.

I believe, like quantum research is demonstrating, that divine life-force energy is a field that can transmit to you, through your Oracle, and can directly affect how you speak, think, act, and feel. I likewise believe that there is a field of energy that extends out from you, to another person, and can directly and powerfully affect how they speak, think, act, and feel. And of course, your own field of energy can directly and powerfully affect how *you* speak, think, act, and feel. So the questions become: Will your field of energy broadcast appreciation or displeasure? And would you like to know how to transmit light?

What You Appreciate, Appreciates

To *appreciate* means to rise in value and to recognize the full worth of, to be grateful for, and to recognize the full implication of something or someone. When you appreciate, you often also feel grateful, and when you feel grateful, you often also feel joyful, pleased, and thankful. Appreciation—naturally linked with gratitude, esteem, and enjoyment—is the counterpart to fearing, faulting, and disparaging that which you listen to and look at. When you practice emitting an appreciative field rather than a critical one, you and others actually rise in value, and everyone's full worth is recognized. I believe that a field of appreciation is a field of divine light, because it allows you to see yourself and others as the Divine sees you: with gratitude, esteem, and enjoyment.

It turns out that whether or not you feel pulled-together, eloquent, and on your A game depends partly on who is listening and the quality of their field. You think that people are what they are; some are beautiful, others are ugly; some are boring, others are interesting. But it turns out that whatever you direct your awareness to will increase and expand. When you direct your awareness to what is beautiful, interesting, or wise about someone (including you), they become even more beautiful, interesting, or wise. When you direct your awareness to what is ugly, boring, or stupid about someone (including you), they will oblige you and become more so.

*what you get
is what you see.*

The same is true for your issues, worries, and problems. You think that when you have a problem, if you focus and work on it, things will get better. But it turns out, although working on your worries has a place, no worry will change until you first deliberately direct your awareness to what you can appreciate about it—what is already good, right, and going well. For example, you might be convinced that if you first get a better wardrobe, clear up your acne, or get asked out on a date, *then* you will feel beautiful and will be able to appreciate yourself. But it turns out that you can appreciate yourself and feel beautiful *right now*, before anything else changes. And it turns out that you *must* shift the way you listen to and look at yourself *first*, in order for an issue, like too few dates, to shift.

> Any gesture of honest and dear seeing toward yourself
> will affect how you experience your world. In fact,
> it will transform how you experience the world.
> **PEMA CHÖDRÖN,** *Comfortable with Uncertainty*

So it turns out that the only things we truly have control over in life are the quality of our fields and to what or whom we are broadcasting them. It turns out that you have incredible power to affect not only how *you* feel, think, act, and how people show up for you, but also to affect how *other people* feel, think, and act, and show up for themselves. By emitting an appreciative field, it is within your grasp to feel attractive, sensuous, and successful even in shitty conditions. By emitting an appreciative field, you become empowered to have almost anyone, anywhere, open their heart to you. And this is also the first step to averting or resolving conflicts, resisting compromises, finding options through impasses, and simply enjoying yourself and your life.

At this point, some people narrow their eyes and look at me critically. (The irony is not lost on me.) They ask if I am simply suggesting that they cover up their judgment and paste on some appreciation. Slap a Band-Aid over the pain of their problems. Because, they tell me, they *feel* their impatience, criticism, trepidation, or disdain. It is the truth of their experience, and to pretend otherwise would be inauthentic.

I am not suggesting you *pretend* or *cover up* anything. Instead, notice the judgment or problem or whatever else, notice your awareness is on it, and then deliberately direct your awareness elsewhere, to something you *can* appreciate. Change the channel you are broadcasting to one of appreciation. Later, if there is still a real issue, there will be room to tune back to the original channel and work out the problem, likely with the fresh perspective, insight, and open-heartedness that appreciation, enjoyment, and gratitude often bring. If you are anything like the women I get to know and get to work with, your default *field* is likely harsh and critical, toward others and toward yourself. I would love for you to retrain yourself to create an appreciative field instead. You can gaze at life through rose-tinted lenses, and your outlook can inspire others to do the same.

Whatever you direct your awareness to will increase and expand. Direct it to how much you suck, you will suck all the more. Direct it to how much you are wonderful, you will be all the more wondrous. It is your choice. I figure, why not choose to see things in their natural glory rather than through the cloudy lens handed to us by a culture that believes women need to be airbrushed in order to be appreciated?

Your illumination is absolutely an inside job. You have the dial. You can feel great about yourself in a world that questions the validity of your existence at every turn. You needn't—and shouldn't—wait for anyone's or anything's approval to feel great about yourself. That is your responsibility and no one and nothing else's.

However, the flip side is that your radiance also blooms when you feel regarded with an appreciative field. When you are noticed for your rightness, just as you are—whether for your body, emotions, ideas, or visions—you will likely feel even more vibrant, vivid, and great about yourself. How you see and how you listen matters. How you are seen and how you are listened to matters.

Let me share with you some of my favorite practices for broadcasting an appreciative field. Don't let their playful or sassy nature fool you. These practices are strenuous meditations that masquerade as blessings; blessings that take shape as fields of appreciation.

APPRECIATION PRACTICE #1 WHEN IN DOUBT, APPRECIATE

You create a field of appreciation simply by changing the channel from bitter and bitchy to caring and curious, so that you can regard what *is* and what is *good* about what is in front of you. Practice this on yourself and on others.

I have found that there are two main ways to practice creating an appreciative field. Try them both.

1 See what *is*, without a tinge of judgment—no right or wrong, good or bad. Just see things as they are, in their *is-ness*.

   This is incredibly liberating and is often enough. For example, instead of harshly proclaiming how you think your friend's dimples make her face look fat and insipid, neutrally notice things as they are: she has dimples.

2 See what *is*, with a positive tinge.

   Imagine that the lens through which you regard the world is appreciation-tinted. Practice seeing people and situations (including yourself) as astonishing, pleasing, true, and wise. In the dimple example, you could notice, positively, the ways your friend's dimples catch and reflect the light, her cheeks lustrous as pearls. You could notice each dimple's curvaceous slope, designed to direct your eye to the mysterious center of each divot.

A great way to get the hang of appreciation is to practice on your own body, perhaps what you see in the mirror. Broadcast an appreciative field, look through the lens of appreciation, and find something about your body that you can appreciate.

Find something that simply *is*, or that is valuable, worthy, wondrous, or sensuous. Remember: appreciate first; find flaws later (if you are still compelled to).

Appreciation is a practice that will teach you to love what you don't even like. What is in front of you might be your friend, your partner, your own reflection, a stranger, some dimples, or a recent heartbreak. When you can see it for what it *is*, not as you wish it to be, its right-ness and beauty will be revealed. And then, a magical thing happens: your bothersome partner, your double chin, that wily stranger, those dimples, or your own complicated life can become resplendent, valu-able, and worthy of gratitude.

Your ability to switch channels—to turn your attention from what is bad and wrong to what simply *is*, to what you can *appreciate*, and to what you can *enjoy*—is an awesome superpower. Your appreciation, of yourself and others, is the special sauce that can take a mundane or miserable moment and make it magical.

APPRECIATION PRACTICE #2   SHAKE IT

Another great way to get the hang of appreciation is to practice on your own *moving* body—as a meditation, a celebration, or a prayer.

Again, power up that ever-handy appreciative field, broadcast it onto your body as well as out into the world, and—shake it.

Shake it! As in, shake what your mama gave you. As in, appreciate what your mama gave you.

Dance, move, wiggle, sashay, prance, sweat, grind, and groove. Take a dance class, do yoga on the beach, or boogie in your own room, all good. Hip-hop, belly dancing, or S Factor are all good. Do it with an instructor or by yourself; do it at home or out in nature—all good.

Like Riya did back in chapter 12, get into your passionate pelvis, your low belly, and *move*. Make it hot, make it holy, make it sweet, make it wrathful. Dance your demons, dance your daemons, dance your aching, dance your wisdom, dance your mystery. Dance like no one is watching you. Dance like everyone is watching you and gets lit up as they do.

Look, as you know, many spiritual and religious traditions say stillness is the best path to inner peace. That seated, quiet contemplation is the ideal way to meet God. As I see it, these practices have been designed by and for the Divine Masculine in all of us. For the Divine Masculine, nothingness is bliss. Yet for the Divine Feminine, the ever-changing, wildly feeling, spiraling, shining everything-of-life is bliss.

Life-force moves. The feminine flavor of God cycles. Feminine Genius spirals, undulates, and fluctuates. Masculine-based spiritual traditions are time honored and have their place. But when a pew or a meditation cushion can't contain the size of your soul, get moving. Shake your booty and turn the other cheek.

Let your moving body be an appreciation and a supplication, all in one.

can i get an amen?
and an ah-woman?

Noticing imperfections can wait. If you slip up and find a fault first, then you owe yourself *three* appreciations. Wait a minute. What? You think there is *nothing* about you to appreciate? I'll have none of that insubordination. That's right, you heard me. Drop and give me *twenty* appreciations!

Appreciate your partner first, then he can show up as trustworthy and sexy. Appreciate your thick thighs first, and then they can be transformed into one of the strongest parts of you. Appreciate the stranger first, and notice as your curiosity (about what might have put her in such a bad mood this morning) relaxes you, and lets you breathe more fully. Appreciate your breakdown first (as your personal invitation from the Queen of the Dark), so your heart can become that much bigger to hold you through the massive challenge.

Appreciation will not only change how you look at yourself and how others listen to you, but it can also become your new default setting. Appreciation is the best antidote to light-dimming conditions like doubts, delusions, people pleasing, and perfectionism. Whether experiencing good or bad times in your life, broadcasting an appreciative field will allow you to see yourself as a freakin' Genius. Self-acceptance will no longer cut it; self-celebration must become the new norm. As my friend Annie would put it, give yourself (internally or out loud) applause, standing ovations, and high-fives for every time you change the channel of your awareness, realize even the most microscopic *aha*s, and do even the tiniest acts of creativity.

And no, you will not become a self-promoting, navel-gazing narcissist. Self-appreciation is not the same as self-aggrandizement. Broadcasting an appreciative field will not tamper with your compassion, lucidity, or motivation—except perhaps to heighten them. You will not lose your ability to lend a hand to others because you are too busy high-fiving yourself.

I promise you, you can love yourself without losing touch with reality. You can do right by someone else *and* yourself at the same time, I swear. In fact, the next practice is all about that.

FROM APPRECIATION TO FLIRTATION

When appreciation drops an octave deeper and richer, it becomes enjoyment. When you are *enjoying* yourself, you are filling yourself with joy like you could fill a pitcher with water. Joy is a feeling of great happiness and pleasure that lets you know you are in contact with something you love and care deeply about. There is a saying in 12-step programs, "A grateful heart doesn't drink." I agree, and add, "A joyful heart doesn't drink—or cut, or binge, or starve, overbook, or overspend." When you are truly experiencing joy, and are truly enjoying yourself, you can't fake it. Joy awakens your truest self, the part of you that is most loving and alive. Your enjoyment puts you automatically and authentically in touch with what moves you, grooves you, and drives you. You become moved, grooved, and driven by delight and abundance, rather than by fear and not-enoughness.

How does flirtation come into this? I define *flirtation* as simply enjoying yourself *at the same time* as enjoying someone or something else. Flirtation is enjoyment, squared. Flirtation winks conspiratorially at you and at the other person, intimating, "I'm kind of great, and you're not so bad yourself!" There are plenty of ways to enjoy yourself while enjoying something or someone else, but one that is especially good for you, as a woman cultivating your light, is flirting.

You can flirt with a baby or a puppy just as well as you can flirt with a hottie in the seat next to you on the bus, or with your partner of twenty years. Flirtation can have platonic or erotic energy. Either way, for those flirtatious moments (and possibly for quite a while afterward), you—and they—are reminded who you truly are. Light and joy return.

One early morning, before flying to guest teach in my friend and colleague's coaching course, I had one such experience of enjoyment, squared. My friend Stacey and I were eating breakfast in a dive diner at a tiny terminal in the San Francisco airport. Now, the list of things I cannot eat is long and makes eating outside my own kitchen an exercise in creativity. It can make me a large pain in the derrière for wait staff worldwide. I ordered, doing my usual routine of "hold this," "add that," and "substitute this for that." As I spoke, I broadcast an invisible but palpable field of appreciation and enjoyment, and directed my awareness to what was right and good about me, and what was right and good about our waiter. Instead of seeing me as an early-morning problem and subtly rolling his eyes, our waiter visibly relaxed and even cracked a grin.

To give you a sense of what a minor miracle this was, let me clarify that it was just past 6:00 a.m. and most everyone at his other tables was grumpy and giving him a hard time. Yet he had smiled when he left our table, a bounce in his step. He even gave us our coffee for free, as we noticed when the bill came. The afterglow of my flirting had extended beyond our meal.

"What were you doing back there?" Stacey asked me as we walked toward our gate. "You were doing something, but I wasn't sure what it was." I explained how I used appreciation fields, and I explained my definition of flirting—my way to enjoy airport food, our waiter, my friend, and myself. As he himself had shared, our waiter was gay, and young enough to be just out of high school. So, my flirting was in no way suggestive or sexual. I was doing the platonic version of creating a field of enjoyment.

"I always figure people don't want to be bothered," Stacey said.

"I used to think that, too," I said. "Sometimes people do just want to be left alone, it's true. But mostly, people are just a heartbeat away from opening up. Given even a tiny window, people can't wait to come out to play."

I don't suggest flirting to get free coffee. Free things are great perks, sure, but even the perks are just a tangible reminder of the generosity that can't help but tumble out of you both. I suggest you flirt to feel full of light, to raise you both in value and worth, and to make you both feel better for the moment you share. Instead of nagging your partner, what if you propose that you will remove one item of clothing for every plate he or she washes from the sink full of yesterday's dinner dishes? Instead of threatening, "If you don't clean up your toys, no dessert for a week!" try putting on music and sharing the new rules of the game: "One gold star sticker for every toy back in the toy chest. And twenty stars equals an extra hour at the pool tomorrow." A moment like that inspires another moment like that. A day full of moments like that, day after day, piles up to life full of light.

You can even flirt—and create a field of enjoyment—without saying much at all or making much eye contact. About three years after working together, I recently asked one of my former clients, Carey, how things were going for her. From the outside, things looked good: her business was growing impressively, and instead of dreading her on-stage appearances, she was enjoying them.

Carey said, "Let me tell you this story that illustrates just how much I have incorporated my sensual energy into my life and how much I feel at home and powerful in my body. A couple of months ago, I was walking through the airport with a little time before my next flight. I was a few pounds over my normal weight, so I wasn't feeling like I was at my best. But I sauntered to my gate, wearing flats and no makeup, feeling happy in my skin, when I saw a tall, handsome Latino man noticing me, quite, shall we say, *appreciatively*? I wasn't in the mood to stop and engage, but I gave him a glance to thank him; and internally, I said to myself, 'That's right. This is what a goddess looks like. Enjoy the view.'"

So, go, goddess, go flirt! Enjoyment, squared, is your next practice.

ENJOYMENT PRACTICE   OPENING UP WITH FLIRTATION

Whether it is done with platonic or erotic intentions, the kind of flirtation I suggest cannot be mistaken for manipulation, misrepresentation, or deceit. It organically brings out your own authenticity and brilliance while bringing them out in another. So, give it a go:

1 Power up your appreciative field and enjoy yourself while enjoying someone or something else.

2 To help get in the right frame of mind, ask yourself internally (or ask your Oracle), "If I direct my awareness to what is right and good about me, and right and good about them, what do I see?" or "What could help this be more enjoyable for me or for them?"

3 With the answers you receive, simply do them, think them, feel them, or say them in the presence of this other person.

As you practice, you will come to see that appreciating someone or something is not only a form of deep enjoyment but is also a gift. Your appreciation, for yourself and for others, is a blessing and a thank you, all in one. Your enjoyment, of yourself and of others, is a field of light.

> Your enjoyment is God's blessing on creation.
> **DR. VICTOR BARANCO**

So, go, goddess. Go flirt with your reflection in the mirror, flirt with your child, flirt with your dancing body, flirt with your partner, flirt with the sunshine, flirt with the woman bundling up your bouquet of flowers. And when she hands you an extra daisy you didn't pay for, give it to the next stranger you see, wrapped in a layer of light.

18

Turning On Your Feminine Genius
Getting Lit Up with Pleasure and Presence

What is to give light must endure burning.
VIKTOR E. FRANKL

Getting lit up—and staying lit up—takes nerve. And verve.

Turning on your light—and keeping it lit—requires the skills of appreciation and enjoyment that you just learned. And it also requires your devotion to *pleasure* and *presence*—two embodied states of being that bring you out of your head and into your body, and bring you powerfully, vividly alive.

Just like a fire can't burn without oxygen, you can't light up or stay lit up without *feeling good* in your body and *staying in* your body. Just like clean, fresh, oxygenated air can let you hear far-off voices as if they were quite close, you will more easily hear your deep desires when you are in a state of pleasure or presence.

You can't hear and heed your Oracle when you manhandle your way through life. Whereas Masculine Genius uses productivity to help you feel good about yourself, Feminine Genius uses pleasure. Whereas Masculine Genius course-corrects through will-powered action, Feminine Genius uses presence. Your entire life will turn out remarkably differently if your default setting is lit up and turned on, embodying your Feminine Genius, rather than jacked up and burned-out, driven by your Masculine Genius.

And so the Feminine Genius kneels at her own altar, lights her own wick, blows on her own flame, and helps it burn brighter.

GETTING LIT UP WITH PLEASURE

> Pleasure is a sensation. It is written into our bodies; it is our experience of delight, of joy. Pleasure will become a marker, a compass pointing to emotional true north.
> **CAROL GILLIGAN,** *The Birth of Pleasure*

Willingly appreciating yourself can be quite a stretch; willfully enjoying your life can be quite radical. But for too many of us, there's nothing quite like the idea (and experience) of *pleasure* to press us against the edge of radical. But as you may remember, the edge of radical is where a woman begins to come alive. So headfirst into pleasure we go.

When your appreciation and enjoyment drop yet another octave deeper and richer, and drop into your sensing, feeling body, the result is a state of pleasure. As I define it, pleasure is a state in which all six of your senses are heightened, not just what you see, hear, smell, taste, and touch, but also what you intuit, desire, and know. Pleasure, a form of erotic energy experienced in and expressed through your body, brings you more sensually alive, intuitively aware, personally confident, and spiritually fulfilled. Pleasure allows you to hear your truth. Pleasure oxygenates your Oracle and stokes your inner fire.

The energy of pleasure, like the energy of Eros, and like a desire, comes in mild, medium, and spicy versions. Mild versions include experiences like cuddling a puppy, smelling the earth after it rains, the aroma of freshly baked chocolate chip cookies, witnessing a random act of kindness, or sensing your body's *yes* or *no*. Medium versions include experiences like the satisfied first-pump of a job well done, jumping off high rocks into a pool of waiting water, reconnecting with a dear friend, the flood of inspiration for a creative project, the hot longing to travel to a new country, or a moment of profound spiritual aliveness. Spicy versions include experiences like the sparks of attraction that fly between you and your lover, your lover's firm grasp on your hips, wanton heavy petting, a soul-opening orgasm, or a soft kiss that melts your knees.

When your body is in a state of pleasure—whether mild, medium, or spicy—you have natural access to your confidence. Confidence allows you to think clearly, choose boldly, and speak your mind freely. When you are feeling confident, you are more connected to your inner knowing; you know "I can do it!" and you know what "it" is. If you hearken back to chapter 12, you will recall the way pleasure in your body stimulates dopamine in your brain, resulting in feelings of motivation, inspiration, and agency.

It might help to imagine the effects of pleasure as similar to the effects of the drug cocaine, a dopamine booster. When they're on cocaine, people feel capable, self-assured, excited, and empowered. But when you are in a state of pleasure, you can *also* feel like a million bucks, with powerful surges of creativity following close behind. Dopamine (although it can be released during stressful experiences as well) is a powerful and natural by-product of pleasurable experiences. For those of us addicted to overusing our Masculine Genius in order to feel capable and powerful, this wisdom about pleasure may seem counterintuitive. But it turns out that tending to the flame of your pleasure actually brings you more truth, clarity, and personal power.

Our Restrictive Beliefs about Pleasure

Now, if you already believe everything I've just said about pleasure, you are a unicorn, and you must write me immediately to tell me your story because it is a far cry from what too many women learn. Over my fourteen years of work with women, I have come to see that our mistrust of pleasure runs deep. We link pleasure with shame. We gorge ourselves on it, and then purge ourselves of it with religious fervor. We believe that going for what feels good is weak, untrustworthy, and disgraceful, and that enjoying ourselves is something we can do only after we have earned it, or only in secret.

Here are some restrictive beliefs about pleasure from a few clients and retreat participants:

- Pleasure is wanton, irresponsible, indulgent, unspiritual, and immoral.

- Pleasure can't be trusted. Pleasure makes people lie and cheat.

- I deserve pleasure only after I have worked hard to earn it.

- If I experience pleasure, there will be less for everyone else.

- If I experience too much pleasure, I will lose control, and people will lose respect for me.

At first, Sian was convinced that cultivating pleasure in her life would be a detour and would make her fall off the wagon. Sian joined my group program because she realized that her lifelong "addictive" behaviors—saying *yes* to too many things and people; doing not what felt right to her, but what she "thought" she should be doing—were exhausting and depleting. She worked for poverty wages, for over ten years, at a nonprofit organization founded by her spiritual teacher. A seasoned member of Alcoholics Anonymous and a seasoned practitioner of selfless, spiritual service, she shared, "The very idea that my strength, wisdom, joy, and nourishment could come from pleasure, rather than self-denial and personal rigor? *What??*"

Zoe, also a participant in my group program, added, "I remember being really young, maybe seven or eight years old, when I learned for certain something I had always suspected: that my dad was with other women. One time when my dad was out of town on a business trip, I was in the dining room with my sisters while my mom called his hotel room and a woman answered the phone. Subconsciously, I decided that pleasure is bad. It is something you lie about. It is something you do in secret, behind your loved ones' backs. It hurts people. For most of my upbringing, I felt lonely and wondered, 'what's the point of being here?'"

You, too, may have come to believe that following pleasure will lead you to pain; but really, it is in *not* following your pleasure that you suffer. It is the banishment and bedevilment of pleasure—the stuffing down of what is native and natural to you—that separates you from you. Without the landmarks of pleasure—your embodied knowing of what you want, what you care about, and what you love—you feel lost.

When I first came to understand the power of pleasure, I was crying myself a river in a weekend course called Basic Sensuality. My then-boyfriend (now husband), Nathan, and I had paid extra to get a private hour-long session with the three workshop leaders, who taught their findings from having lived for over forty years in a collective living experiment called More University.

At the time, Nathan and I had been together for three rocky years, and we needed some help with a true impasse in our relationship—whether or not to have a child together. Nathan was a *no*; I was pretty sure I was a *yes*. At minute fifty-five, one of the teachers stopped us and said, "Look, I don't know if you should have a child or not. It's a lot of work. I love my kid, but it is hard to pull it off well. But what I do know is that you are having a miserable time figuring it out. What if you had a pleasurable time figuring it out?"

A pleasurable time? Finding our way through such a serious stand-off? The gears of my brain ground to a halt. Smoke poured out of my ears as I tried to compute what the teacher was suggesting. *Enjoy* this wrenching process? Could that be done? Should that be done? I took a walk by myself along the one-lane road into town. As I walked, I realized how easy it was for me to fall into tears, despair, and shame when things got difficult. Under pressure, my go-to was self-doubt, followed by helplessness, followed by blame. But what if amid the stresses and storms that life inevitably throws at us all, I could just as easily reach for pleasure?

I then had to admit how addicted I was to having a crappy experience while working out big things. I couldn't even separate "working out big things" from "crappy experience," they were so conjoined in my mind. In fact, was I a woman who was actually *able* to be happy—sustainably happy? Like Snow White, I was waiting for someone to awaken me; like Cinderella, I was expecting that something else would sweep in and make my life great. I was a happiness sieve, constantly leaking. There, in the presence of roadside springtime daffodils, I came to the realization that I was actually *very* interested in gaining ownership of my pleasure, joy, and quality of life.

So, I got practicing. I took on pleasure. In the next few months, I would ask myself, over and over each day, "How can I make this moment more pleasurable for myself?" I would listen to the answers, the often-strange answers, which bubbled up from my body and my psyche (I didn't know about my Oracle back then, so I wasn't consulting her), and I followed them.

Instead of always working late until 6:00 or 7:00 p.m. every evening, I would take one day a week to stop working in the afternoon and go get a massage, one of my favorite ways to get back in my body and feel sensually alive. I set a reminder on my computer so I would remember to take a dance break at various times during the day, shaking my booty to a song I loved. I mustered all my resolve and said *no* to things that felt like obligations, so I could arrive at the end of the day with energy left for quality sex and quality conversation with my partner. I wrote, "You are gorgeous!" with a dry-erase marker on the bathroom mirror and smiled at the compliment every time I saw it. I picked out dresses in indigo and vermillion, leaving my all-black outfits in the back of my closet. I left an extra dollar tip for the barista, just to see a little light creep across her sleepy face.

It was less about the actions I took, however, and more about how I *felt* each time I chose to invoke pleasure. I felt sassy, supple, and strong. Generous. Nourished. Intuitive. Sure-footed. True. I grew a calm yet vibrant center within myself that I could access on good days as well as bad.

From time to time, Nathan and I would revisit the baby question. As it turned out, his *no* was more because he could see that having an infant (although an absolute influx of divine love) would be rather stressful, a perfect storm for burnout, a perfect recipe for divorce. I understood that Nathan was less of a *no* to the actual experience of having and raising a child together, and more of a *no* to losing the joyful, playful me, because of my default collapse when faced with challenges.

We both started to cherish this new side of me: A me that could have a good time, regardless of circumstances. A me that could be happy without a reason. A me that quite possibly could stay lit up and turned on, even amid the stressful storms of new motherhood. As of this writing, our son is five years old.

From all this, I realized that increasing the pleasure in my body and in my life was essential to my well-being—and to the survival of my marriage. It is what Sian and Zoe realized as well, back in my mentorship program. After devoting herself to her pleasure in this way, Sian could no longer link spiritual service with suffering. On the advice of her Oracle, she quit her job, an agonizing but ultimately liberating choice. She told me recently that every Monday is "me day" and she leaves it free for self-care and time with women friends. Sian is careful of her knee-jerk reaction to cram her schedule. "As I am saying no to more things, I am saying yes to my inner little girl, yes to my true self," she smiles. At the time I wrote this chapter, Sian—a year after quitting her stressful job—had just started her new job as a coach in a fast-growing company with a generous salary. And Mondays off, naturally.

I checked in with Zoe many years after our work together. She just had her first baby. "Putting attention on pleasure has been life or death for me. It is all about coming alive again. Yes, life feels tedious and hard sometimes, but it doesn't have to be that way all the time. Instead of wondering why I'm here, I feel like I *get to be* here. It is important for me to remember that in every moment I have a choice. It takes a lot of courage and effort for me to not revert back to the default belief that pleasure is bad. But when I am feeling stressed, and I am able to stop and ask myself, 'How can I experience more pleasure in this moment?' it can be kind of a game-changer." For Zoe and for all of us, pleasure helps our power flow.

> A woman's power is directly proportional to the amount of pleasure she is experiencing in her life.
> **CALLAN LYNNE**

The Pleasure Question

The question, "How can I make this moment more pleasurable for myself?" is one that Zoe and Sian—as well as my clients, friends, participants—have learned to ask all day, every day. For them, as for me, it has become a reflex, like blinking. The pleasure question will change your entire experience of being a woman, if you use it. And it will bring out your Feminine Genius, if you let it.

Let's break the pleasure question down a bit.

What do I mean by "pleasurable"?

Pleasure is a widening of any or all of your six senses—what you see, hear, touch, taste, smell, and intuit—so you *feel more*. What brings you pleasure will be very different from what brings me pleasure. This question gets you into research mode: What really does it for you?

For example, if your friend were to ask the pleasure question, she might get an answer such as, "Put on music and belt it out." Whereas *you* might get an answer such as, "Take a bath." And *I* might get an answer such as, "Buy a sandwich and give it to that homeless girl." What lights you up will be totally distinct from what lights me up, from what lights your friend up. As it should be.

And what moment do I mean by "this moment"?

I suggest asking the pleasure question during boring, crappy, or "meh" moments, such as when you are waiting in line at the grocery store, on hold with customer service, in an argument with a friend, or stuck in traffic. It can help you breathe fresh life into mundane moments and aggravating situations.

I also suggest asking the pleasure question during times when you are already relatively lit up and turned on, like during good sex, a fascinating theatre production, or a great party. It is radical to know that even when things are good, you can turn the dial up to great. (For the really tough times, I have a different practice for you a little later in this chapter.) I know it might feel counterintuitive to *enjoy* rush hour traffic, and audacious to ask, "This ecstatic lovemaking is amazing, but what if it was even *more* pleasurable?" But this is what I am asking you to imagine—and practice.

Now, the last part, "for myself"?

Wait, wait, wait. You might be wondering if I am really sure I mean that last part, right? "Isn't it selfish," you might be thinking, "to increase my pleasure solely for myself? What about everyone else? Are you lauding narcissism and greed, encouraging me to just get mine and snub everyone else in the process? Instead of the pleasure question, is this actually the 'enjoy myself and stick it to those suckers' question?"

Nope.

But most of us have these valid concerns because we misunderstand the power—and the natural impulses—of a lit up and turned on woman. There is a saying, "If Mama ain't happy, ain't nobody happy." You probably have firsthand experience with this saying, either with your mother, as a mother yourself, or, well, around pretty much any woman.

Asking the pleasure question is like putting your own oxygen mask on first. A woman who cultivates her light in these ways is in her most natural state, which is one of generosity, compassion, confidence, and grace. When you are devoted to pleasure, you naturally have plenty of awareness to direct to the people you love and care about. When you are less blinded by self-doubt and chronic overwhelm, you have greater capacity to see what could truly make a difference for them.

In this world that is both anti-pleasure and pro-productivity—and that espouses unconscious consumption—devoting yourself to your pleasure is radical, yet imperative. A go-go-go lifestyle pumps adrenaline and cortisol (stress hormones) into your body so that you experience low-grade stress and anxiety, day in and day out. This can make for weight gain, hormone disruption, fatigue, insomnia, mood swings, blood sugar dips, irritability, moodiness, inflammation, and depression.

When you are stressed-out and burned-out, your body is more concerned with *surviving* than with *thriving*. In survival mode, all your bandwidth goes to outrunning a tiger or sprinting toward heaven, regardless of what form the *tiger* or *heaven* comes in. When you are simply surviving, there's too much "static" in your system for you to actually hear messages from your Oracle trying to get a word in edgewise. Look, I am all for getting stuff done. I am all for productivity and focus and the high that comes from them. It is just that most of us, men and women alike, rely on these Masculine Genius strengths to the detriment of our Feminine Genius strengths—and big, bad imbalances can result.

Pleasure isn't synonymous with *indulging* and *doing nothing*, even though most of us could do with a lot more bliss and replenishment in our lives. Being in a state of pleasure allows something deep within you to relax. An aspect of your Genius becomes available. You connect the dots. You feel self-possessed. You have foresight and larger vision. You feel like you're having a great time. You feel blessed and on fire. You can clearly hear your Oracle—your *yes*es and *no*s, your desires, and your next steps.

Might you make others uncomfortable if you are having too good a time? Might you disappoint? Might you feel lonely as you swim upstream while the collective culture is caught in the status quo? Maybe. But I am absolutely clear that the point of your life is *not* to turn down your light in order to uphold a sense of propriety in a system that is beyond broken. The point of your life is to burn brightly with integrity and care, to shine your light through the dark so we can all find our way home.

So here is my best practice for lighting your candle, bowing, and entering devotedly into the dojo called pleasure.

PLEASURE PRACTICE #1   THE PLEASURE QUESTION

1   At least once a day, or as often as womanly possible, ask yourself (or your Oracle) the following question: "How can I make this moment more pleasurable for myself?"

2   And then do, say, think, or feel what you hear.

3   Rinse and repeat. Enjoy.

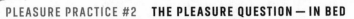

PLEASURE PRACTICE #2   THE PLEASURE QUESTION — IN BED

For your spicy, sensual, sexual experiences, this practice is meant to call your awareness away from worry and distraction, back into the here and now, your six senses, your desires, your Oracle, and your body.

1   Ask yourself (or your Oracle) the pleasure question during your sexual experiences, whether by yourself or with another. Use the pleasure question to direct your awareness to what you are *feeling*, rather than what you are *thinking*. It can work wonders.

2   Then do, say, think, or feel what you hear. Enjoy!

It is easy to get distracted by racing thoughts during sensual situations. Notice yourself thinking things such as, "I can't relax, there are dishes to be done." "Do I look good from this angle?" "Will he make a good father?" "Will the neighbors hear?" Then instead, *feel* your way to your pleasure, to your lover's pleasure, to each of your lovely senses.

Try using your thoughts to attend to what you are *feeling*. For example, you can redirect the worry, "Will the neighbors hear?" to noting your feelings such as, "Shivers all the way to my toes." "The tender touch of her upper lip on mine." "A ripple of warmth over my chest." "I feel shy and like a lioness at the same time."

Honor your feelings. Note them. Grow them. Widen them. Expand them. Deepen them. Adore them. Thank them.

The Divine is pleased when you take pleasure from what she sends your way. Life itself gets happy when you enjoy it. Your Oracle cheers, and Feminine Genius applauds when you say thank you.

Let your pleasure be a prayer. Let the mundane become mystical. When it comes to your light, you mustn't tone it down. Burn hotter.

GETTING LIT UP WITH PRESENCE

> The deeper that sorrow carves into your
> being, the more joy you can contain.
> **KAHLIL GIBRAN, *The Prophet***

Getting lit up—and staying lit up—isn't always *happy, happy, joy, joy*.

When it comes to cultivating your inner light, sometimes it is not pleasure that is called for, but *presence*—a state of being that brings you into your body and into the now, with veracity and often ferocity. Some situations require you to ask not, "How can I make this moment more pleasurable for myself?" but instead, "How can I come more alive in this moment? How can I be most true? How can I be fully *here*? How can I be fully *me*?" Even when enjoying yourself doesn't seem like an option, showing up with presence always is. The more present you are, the more clearly you can hear your truth, the less likely you are to respond with knee-jerk reactions, and the more you will feel at home in your body.

Presence helps unhook you from restrictive beliefs. Presence is oxygen for Oracles. Presence reconnects you to the wisdom of the collective soul. It is intoxicating, enlivening, and healing. It allows you to be here now, and to be *you* now. Because your big brain might like to pretend it's the boss, and because your days are so demanding and your past so painful, cultivating presence takes some practice.

There are all kinds of tough situations—yep, another freakin' growth opportunity—that will tempt you to "leave your body," *will* your way through, or go lifeless, reactive, or numb. Your plan for a natural, pleasurable labor will fall apart. The baby will cry moments after you put him down, not caring that you have not slept more than three hours in a row in over six months. You will feel so low that you will not know how to get out of bed in the morning. Your lover will walk out of the room while you're in midsentence, while your heart is open, and you will want to throw daggers and do damage. You will be on the dance floor at the wedding reception, loving the song but feeling like a dork, wanting to slink off to the bathroom. Your life will be good, with all kinds of things to be grateful for, but you will still feel a piercing longing for something more. And yet, in the moments you least want to be asked, and in the moments you least think you can do it, Feminine Genius will ask you, *So, sweet one, who are you, truly? Instead of running off to hide, shrink, push, bare your claws, or go lifeless, will you stay with me here in your body?*

As I see it, you leave your body and the present moment because you don't want to feel so bad, or feel so much. So the leaving, willing, clawing, or numbing through whatever method is your favorite works. It helps you to not feel so darn much. But as you feel less of the present moment, you also feel less of yourself. As you feel less of your dark, you also feel less of your light. So, lovely, as you begin to thaw, turn yourself on and come more fully to life; as you feel more joy, you may also feel more sorrow. It is a hazard—I mean blessing—of walking the path of Feminine Genius.

So, for the next sorrowful, tough times, the practice I favor is The Grounding Rod.

A grounding rod (or lightening conductor) is usually a tall metal pole or object that is mounted onto a building, ship, or even a tree. As the tallest object around, it will attract lightening—the high-wattage electrical current in the air. The grounding rod collects the electricity into itself, and then literally *grounds* the energy by running it through the rod and then into the physical earth. Should lightening hit, it will get routed right into the ground instead of completely frying the building, ship, or tree.

When electricity strikes in your life, your body can be the grounding rod, running the intense energy right into the earth so that you can feel fully present instead of feeling completely fried.

PRESENCE PRACTICE   THE GROUNDING ROD

This grounding rod somatization (a visualization that you feel in your body) is incredibly useful for staying present and grounded in your body, and resourceful even in challenging emotional situations, without numbing out, blowing out, or shutting down.

1   Imagine your spine as a rod, collecting any intense energy that might be coming *at* you or coming from *within* you.

2   Imagine moving the energy down your spine, down your legs, through your feet, and finally into the ground.

3   For extra gold stars, imagine that the intense sensations are *charging up* your Oracle, like charging up a battery, as they make their way through your body, down your spine, and into the ground. What remains, after you have run the emotional current into the ground, is *presence*—bright, true presence.

4   You can then ask yourself, "If I don't have to knee-jerk my way through this moment, what other options just might be available right now?" Or "What would my Oracle do?"

Your state of presence reconnects you to the most brilliant parts of yourself and lets *those* parts choose what step to take next. That next step will not always be the easiest, quickest, or most obvious one, but it will always be the truest one, and it will always be the one that brings with it the most life-force.

The grounding rod welcomes you back to the present moment, and presence welcomes you back to life.

Because, at the end of the day, do you want to *be here* for your life—all of it—or do you want to duck for cover and miss it? Masculine Genius does what needs to be done by letting you numb to your body and feelings. Feminine Genius does what needs to be done by getting you fully present to your body and feelings. Which is, ironically, kind of a pleasure.

LIT UP AND TURNED ON: YOUR OPTIMAL SETTING

> For your body, being "turned on" is simply
> another version of "being alive" without any
> hint of right or wrong associated with it.
> **JENA LA FLAMME**

Cultivating your light takes pleasure and presence. Like a candle, when you are burned-out and dimmed down, you feel stuck, unlit, and opaque. There is no current of power running through your body or your life. Lit up and turned on, however, you feel powerful, radiant, and lucid. You conduct light. You and the source of your light are one.

Turned off by the term *turned on*? It is provocative on purpose. Other women have used *joyful, happy, delighted, pleasured, vibrant, balanced, alive, peaceful, "full-body yes," confident, energized, inspired, excited, illuminated,* and *activated.* Call it what you will. I call it your light.

I provoke you on purpose because your very life is at stake. Really. Here's what I mean: Imagine or recall a moment when you were quite stressed-out or burned-out. Perhaps anxious, overwhelmed, resourceless, depleted, go-go-go, bitchy, or on autopilot. Really feel it.

In this stressed-out, burned-out state, what is your outlook like? How do you do the stuff that needs to get done in your life? What do you believe to be true about yourself? Others? The world? Life? Imagine having a difficult conversation in this state. How might it go?

In contrast, now imagine yourself in a lit-up and turned-on state, feeling powerful, radiant, and lucid. And then check: Which version of you—burned-out or turned-on—feels more like your most aligned self? Which would you prefer as your default setting? Which would you trust the most to make an important choice? Which feels more empowered? Which is most flexible? Which is most connected to your inner knowing? Which version would you like to *be* when your partner texts you to break up with you, when your car stops working, or when you are planning your goals for the year? Which version of you would you like to wake up with each morning?

The masculine path of awakening is often defined by agony, asceticism, deprivation, and regimentation; but the feminine path requires pleasure, enjoyment, appreciation, and embodied presence.

When you are numbed out, you cannot accurately hear your inner guidance. When you are turned on, you are a clear channel. When you are dimmed down, others might look right past you. When you are turned on, they cannot take their eyes off you. When you are burned-out, your life-force ebbs and you feel sick, sad, mad, and off-course. When you are turned on, each step along your path brings you more powerfully alive.

When she came to work with me, Lynn decidedly *did not* feel lit up or turned on. She was unable to get out of her five-year toxic relationship with Jay—a man who was deceptive and elusive—even though she knew she wanted to and needed to. Only with Jay, it seemed, did Lynn's body and soul come alive in profound ways. She felt that he was the source of her light and fire and zest for life, and so he became a habit nearly impossible to quit.

It's true that when people get in touch with their light through a new situation or exciting lover—something outside of themselves—they can get addicted. It can feel as profound as finding the elixir of life after a long slog through the underworld. As you have seen in the news countless times, and maybe in your friends' lives, too, they may risk their careers, public image, marriages, and friendships for the connection.

Lynn and I worked on her "addiction" head-on for about four months. She practiced getting in touch with her Oracle and desires, and then grew the courage and skill to express what she truly wanted with Jay. When she could see that he was not able to adjust or step up to the levels of honesty and commitment she wanted and needed, she was able to begin detoxing from him, and was ultimately able to let him go completely. It felt far from easy, but it felt absolutely true. She finally began to see herself as everyone around her saw her: a woman who was vibrant, beautiful, kind, financially successful, physically fit, and full of life, a woman that any man would feel fortunate to be with.

Just before the end of our program together, Lynn told me that an old childhood friend, Nick, had tracked her down on Facebook. Reconnected with her sense of herself as beautiful and whole, devoted to her inner light, and emboldened to speak her truth, Lynn quit a harmful habit named Jay and left some space for a new and wonderful one. She realized her light was not dependent on her lover; it was her own. And only after claiming that could Nick come into her life. At the time I was writing this chapter, Lynn emailed me a photo of her and Nick at their wedding.

The most choice & power appear when you are lit up

Your resting pulse is feeling turned on. Your default setting. Your birthright.

It is not *fine*. It is not *okay*. It is not *life's a bitch and then you die*. It is joy. The lustrous pleasure of being alive. Each of your five senses drenching you. Feeling free in your skin. Knowing what you know. Feeling what you feel. Saying audaciously, "You know, screw these zits and the ten new pounds and my abandonment issues and that I just got dumped and that I just spilled coffee on my new dress. Screw all that because you know, right now, if I'm really honest, I feel pretty grand. In fact, I am one hot number. Holy light shines from these eyes. It feels good to swing these hips and toss this hair and let this knowing smile illuminate the whole neighborhood."

Feeling turned on has essentially nothing to do with you having the perfect body, weight, shoes, partner, house, job, or lipstick color. Feeling turned on is an inside job, even though—*wowza!*—from the outside, we experience you as a full-wattage supernova.

Relocating your light in these ways can be like coming back to life after ten years in a coma. It can be like regaining the use of your arms after a paralysis, suddenly able to swim, bake cookies, run your fingers through your hair, and hug your grandmother. When your Feminine Genius is turned on, you are sovereign, beholden to no one, and—á la the temple priestesses and virgins—can't be easily controlled. You are just as likely to eschew the status quo in your relationships, sexuality, religion, spirituality, voting, buying, communicating, parenting, and investing. Your light is the ultimate high, the ultimate relief, and the ultimate freethinking elixir.

The stark raving madness of this world only intensifies when we refuse to think for ourselves and refuse to like ourselves. I mean, if we were all in a passionate love affair with ourselves, would we buy the snake oil? If we were all busy gettin' busy with Shakti, would we subject ourselves to a suffocating job or relationship? Would we go to war with ourselves in an effort to fit in? It is threatening to any status quo system to have a woman own her light. And it can also be potentially dangerous to the woman who rediscovers her light. Let me explain.

I urge you to resist acting like a junkie fixated on what seems to be the source of this magic potion of life, be it a new lover, course, practice, food, or pair of shoes. There are likely underlying issues that your newly found (or rediscovered) light may temporarily blind you from seeing.

Don't get confused. *You* are the owner of your light. The lover, the flirtation, the course, the practice, the shoes: they help. But the source of your light is within you, infinitely renewable. Or, more accurately, you lease your light from the Sacred Feminine by being born in a woman's body. It is your sacred responsibility to become a black-belt badass when wielding your light. Otherwise, it's like getting a sharpened samurai sword for your third birthday. Ouch. Don't forget.

You may have thought that the *less* you focus on your bodily pleasure in your workaday life, and the *more* you try to stay present on your meditation cushion, the closer you will get to enlightenment. But really, the path of Feminine Genius asks you to wake up and see that you are already a source of light.

Lit up and turned on: what a shameless way to live and love, to work and work out, to mother and lead, to communicate and meditate, to feel and be.

when your Feminine Genius is Turned on you will light and lead our world

19

Activating Your Receiver

Are You Pickin' Up What the Divine Is Puttin' Down?

> Until we can receive with an open heart, we are
> never really giving with an open heart. When we
> attach judgment to receiving . . . we knowingly
> or unknowingly attach judgment to giving . . .
> **BRENÉ BROWN,** *The Gifts of Imperfection*

The world—and countless people in it—cannot wait to conspire with you to help you meet your desires and cannot wait to gift you with blessings.

can you imagine that?

There is something wildly potent and much needed that is asking to get into this world through you. The quantum field, the collective soul, your Feminine Genius is, right now, like a radio broadcasting your next inspiration to you.

can you hear it?

Roaming loose through the world there is a force for truth, beauty, and creativity wanting to welcome you into your life, imprint itself into your body, and planning to work you, change you, and mold you into the woman you are aching to become.

can you let it in?

If you are like most women and get squirmy about *receiving*, then your answer to each of these questions is likely *no*. I too was squirmy for most of my life, and, at the beginning of our work, most of my clients and participants are as well.

To *receive*, in the *gift* sense, means to be given, to be presented with, or to accept delivery of something, such as a gift or an offering.

To *receive*, in the *radio* sense, means to detect, to pick up, or to be a receptacle for a signal or a broadcast.

To *receive*, in the *hostess* sense, means to greet, to welcome, and to take in, such as a houseguest, communion, or confession.

How else are you—like a light bulb—to illuminate, except by first *receiving* the electric energy that then becomes light?

ACTIVATING YOUR RECEIVER

There are a good many reasons you—like so many women—might discount the power of receiving and (purposely or accidentally) deactivate your receiver. You may think that receiving means you have to take everything that is offered, hook, line, and sinker. Or you think that you don't deserve what is offered. Or you *expect* or feel *entitled* to what you want, and thereby conflate your grabbing and grasping with receiving. Or you believe that receiving will turn you into a charity case, and you do not want to be perceived as incapable or undependable.

Additionally, you may think that if you accept help or support, you will "owe" whoever has helped or supported you, and you do not want to be in anyone's debt. You might associate receiving with a loss of power and control, or an inability to protect yourself. Perhaps when you have received in the past, others got angry or envious. You might also doubt that there is enough to go around, so if you receive, you fear you will therefore rob someone else. You could fear that the world and the people in it are inherently indifferent or malicious, and therefore dangerous to rely on or receive from. And perhaps most surprisingly, receiving can confront you with the wonderful and uncomfortable truth that you are powerful and worth giving to.

Receiving, whether in the form of help, money, a compliment, a desire, a vision, or a gift, might make you feel out of control. You feel reprehensible, guilty, greedy, and bad. So when you refuse to receive, you adopt the strategy of giving, giving, and giving, and feel the relief that comes from feeling in control. You feel virtuous, innocent, helpful, and good. However, when you elevate giving and demote receiving, you unwittingly remove yourself from the universal cycle of give-and-take. You limit your ability to hear your own truth and become unable to be positively affected by life and your fellow human beings. Activating your receiver is a healthy challenge to all these assumptions.

Shortly after relocating to San Francisco from New York City, I was at a dinner party at the home of some new friends. Glass of cold white wine in hand, waiting for the hot tub to warm up and the kale-and-quinoa appetizers to be ready (ah, California livin'), I cruised my hosts' bookshelves and ran across a book titled *Pronoia* by Rob Brezsny. The book is fantastically fantastical, devoted to a concept that Brezsny coined, which is essentially the opposite of paranoia.

During my twelve years as an East Coaster, I became intimate with the concept of paranoia, which means that you believe that the world and the people in it are out to get you. If that is your worldview, as it is for many women no matter where they live, it makes good sense to give the finger to receiving. My own paranoia took the form of perfectionism, as it does for many women. I assumed that the world, and the people in it, just couldn't wait to sink their teeth into me. So becoming perfect, in body, speech, and in action, would protect me, I thought, against anyone finding fault with me, hurting me, or rejecting me, ever.

In contrast, *pronoia* says that the Universe is conspiring to shower you with blessings. I had to stop and consider: What might my life be like if I knew that I lived in a world that not only adored me but was also listening intently to what I wanted? What might change if I knew that I lived in a land that simply couldn't wait for the next opportunity to bathe me in milk and honey?

After the dinner party and the discovery at the bookshelf, I allowed the concept of pronoia to become more than a nifty idea, to totally saturate me, body and soul, and to become my new worldview. Over a few months, I started to assume that the energy of life was good-natured, and operated like benevolent gnomes, genies, or fairies that hid behind trees and in my mailbox, in anticipation of sending me little bolts of joy, placing gifts in my path, directing me to fabulous parking spots, and otherwise demonstrating how much the world loved me, wanted me in it, and wanted the best for me. For me as well as everyone else.

The idea of pronoia helped me see that people are mostly kind, and that when they are judgmental or mean, it has more to do with the wounds they are nursing or the hard rows they are hoeing, and nearly nothing to do with me. And that, given half a chance, people are just dying to open up, light up, and reveal their magnificent hearts to me. I started to see that in my hands was the key to feeling safe, happy, and held in my own world, and having other people feeling safe, happy, and held when they were with me.

Without receiving, you can't let in the important stuff—like love, raises, acclaim, care packages, fairy magic sprinkles, and guidance about your next move in life. But when your paradigm becomes pronoia, receiving starts to seem like a really good idea.

You might assume that to receive you must become passive, but this is not the case. Receiving may be the Feminine Genius juxtaposition to the Masculine Genius strength of actively "making shit happen," but there is nothing passive about receiving. Receiving actually requires your intention and willing participation. You do not have to get your PhD in doormat and let whatever or whoever walk all over you in order to become a great receiver.

Becoming a great receiver helps you re-understand that your needs, wants, and desires are not repulsive but are in fact some of the most wildly attractive forces in the world. The skill of receiving is an important step in literally attracting to you that which you want. While your Masculine Genius *executes* and *acts*, your Feminine Genius *attracts* and *magnetizes*. By activating your receiver, you draw things toward you and let them in.

Receiving is also trustable and generous. It is the opposite of selfish. How else do others get to give their gifts if they are prohibited from contributing to you? Although you may think that asking for help will make you burdensome, consider what happens inside others whom you ask for help. They step out of their own life dramas and troubles, if even for a moment. As they help you, they show up as capable, wise, proactive, and present, even if moments before they may have been feeling overwhelmed, bored, or sorry for themselves.

One of the abilities that engenders the most trust and respect between people, says the researcher and writer Brené Brown, is the ability not only to *give* support but also to *ask for* and *receive* support. Activating your receiver allows you, like a light bulb, to give and receive light. And you have a golden receiver, right within your body: your Oracle. Your Oracle is like a radio antenna, or as I prefer to describe it, your Oracle is your direct line to the Divine, getting signals, loud and clear, expressly for you and your Feminine Genius path. Allowing Feminine Genius to signal to you, give to you, nourish you, and shape you is the ultimate act of trust and strength, not of weakness. Turning on your receiver might take some practice. And so, let's practice.

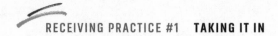

RECEIVING PRACTICE #1   TAKING IT IN

1   Imagine a dear friend giving you a genuine compliment.

2   Imagine her words entering your body like a morsel of delicious food, or a beautiful scent, or a color you love.

3   Imagine tasting her words and the intention behind her words. Savor them. Chew. Taste. Swallow. Imagine the compliment being absorbed into your bloodstream, nourishing and strengthening you.

4   If the scent or color metaphor resonates more with you, fully breathe in her words and the intention behind them. Imagine them imprinting you, like drops of colored ink saturating a glass of clear water. Imagine them wafting through you, like the smell of newly cut grass, fresh and delicious.

5   Let her words add to you, change you, feed you, and affect you. You may even want to imagine the energy of her compliment nourishing and "charging up" your Oracle, like recharging a battery.

6   If you're practicing this in real time, I recommend these responses:
    • "Thank you, it's true."
    • "Thank you, I receive that happily (or fully)."
    • "Thank you, I accept."

You can apply this practice to more than just a friend's kind words. You can practice this with all manner of things you are offered, such as physical gifts, a smile from a stranger, or the sensations you feel from a lover's touch. And with things that are just hanging out in your world waiting for you to receive them, like sunshine, birdsong, a scent drifting by, or a hot bath. Or things you want to attract to you, such as a right-fitting partner, a new mentor or teacher, or clarity on a new direction for your work.

"THANK YOU, IT'S TRUE"

Okay, it is good not to gloss over this one: "Thank you, it's true." Inspired from my mentor Regena, who shared it with me on the steps of her brownstone many years ago, this simple, bold phrase has never left me. If you feel your cheeks flush with discomfort at the thought of responding thusly to an incoming compliment—good. Do it anyway. We women are overtrained to deflect, play humble, and self-efface at any chance we get, but especially when we are praised or are about to get something we actually want and have worked hard for. Self-appreciation is not the same thing as narcissism, although women are notoriously confused about this fact. The bearer of the compliment is just stating the truth of what they see or feel. Give them—and yourself—the respect of acknowledging that truth. Allow yourself to shine.

If this is still a sticky point for you, imagine for a moment that you find the perfect gift for someone you love. Maybe it's in a tucked-away store you have never before been in. You know that it is just what your friend has been wanting, so you buy it, flushing with pleasure as you do. You wrap it carefully in beautiful paper, and decorate it with little paste-on jewels and handwritten words that are meaningful to your friend. Then imagine yourself heady with anticipation in front of your friend, holding out the lovingly created gift. And then imagine your friend shutting down, turning away, and saying, "I couldn't possibly. I don't deserve that."

That is what we women do daily to love, gifts, appreciation, praise, and our deep desires (that we are busy working our asses off for but are too well trained in deflection to actually receive). Instead of giving the finger to the pronoiacally inclined Universe, and all the gnomes, fairies, genies, daemons, and loving people in it, remember that receiving is far from selfish. It is actually honoring and empowering.

Here's an example of how important it is to receive. I have never met my client Vanessa face to face, but over the phone, her voice is surprisingly deep and resonant. One morning, she shared with me how she'd benefited from one of my online courses: "I have struggled most of my life with being in my head and disconnected from my body and spent a lot of my life being numb, not allowing myself to feel the good because I didn't want to feel the bad. I used your course the first time to call in my life partner. I benefited so much that I immediately repeated it, and I met my partner two weeks into my second round."

Vanessa went on: "I started by somaticizing and feeling the possibility of him out there somewhere, wanting to be with me as much as I wanted to be with him. I felt that I had always blocked myself somehow from having what I truly want in a relationship. I realized that I hadn't been open to accepting this. The course really helped me open up, recognize when it was coming to me, and allow myself to have it. From the very first time I met him (now my partner for over two years) and every day since then, I say to the Universe, 'Thank you, I accept.' Both he and I had done a lot of other 'work' to be ready for our relationship, but I know that the final step for me was clearly seeing the beliefs I had that blocked by ability to receive. It feels powerful. Truly amazing."

Vanessa opened herself to receive, to beautiful effect. But being open to receive a partner also has another meaning I want to share with you. The number one thing that our *partners* want most in intimacy is to feel accepted, seen, and known. Women who are used to giving but not receiving often block the ability to truly *receive* a partner and to have their beloved partner feel accepted, seen, known—rather than held away at a safe distance.

This is a tragedy that can be averted or reversed with your skillful practice of receiving. Even if it is a physical gift or actual words, it is really *energy* that you are receiving. So whether the thing to be received is physical or emotional, animate or inanimate, already here or about to be here, draw it toward you, receive it, and let it nourish you. Magnetize it to you. Let it come to you. Take it in.

But, hold on a moment. What about when you don't actually *want* the offer, the phone number, the ogling, or the gift that's coming your way? What about when you are *not* looking to call in a partner at all, but a guy comes up to you at a party, gives you a stunning compliment, and hands you his number on a cocktail napkin? What about when the construction worker catcalls as you walk by? What about when your aunt Edna wants to bring by a fresh tuna noodle casserole, and you don't eat gluten or large deep-sea fish? What about when your mama wants to give you a third helping of mashed potatoes at dinner, and you are stuffed? Then, you say *yes* to the *intention*, while you say *no* to the offering.

There are going to be times when you do not want your receiving channel open at all. It is more than okay to take down your antenna part way or all the way. Here's one way to practice that.

RECEIVING PRACTICE #2   THANK YOU, BUT NO

Try out these sentences—and improvise your versions thereof:

- For Aunt Edna situations: "I really feel your care and the attention you put into making this for me (offering this to me), but I can't accept."
- For cocktail party instances: "You seem like a man that fully appreciates the power and beauty of women. Thank you, but no."
- For Mama's mashed potatoes circumstances: "These are wonderful; I can taste the love in them, but no thank you. I'm full. I've got exactly the right amount."
- For the construction worker's whistles: skip to Receiving Practice #3.

TO RECEIVE OR NOT TO RECEIVE

Remember Violette who has often wondered what to do with the intensity of her feelings instead of, as she put it, screaming like her hair is on fire? Violette's receiving channel is naturally so wide open that she is often on the verge of tears or ecstasy, feeling the depth and intensity of her own emotions, those of her friends and colleagues, and also that of the collective human (woman) experience. Often, she stops whatever she is in the middle of, and—unable to do much of anything else for a while—lies down, allowing it all to pierce her to her bones.

However, for Violette, being able to adjust *when* she receives, *what* she receives, and *how much* she receives—so as not to be always knocked over and totally incapacitated from the sheer magnitude of it all—has been a gift.

Here is a version of what has helped Violette.

RECEIVING PRACTICE #3 TO RECEIVE OR NOT TO RECEIVE?

It is as important to be able to take something in as it is to say "No, thank you" and keep that something out. And, it is also important that *when* you let it in, you have a say about *how much* you let in. These are two powerful somatizations (visualizations you feel in your body) so you can have choices, and begin to conduct the energy of what you receive. Try them both and see which works best for you.

THE CELL MEMBRANE

Think back to biology class for a moment and recall how cell walls in the bodies of living organisms work. Cell walls are the layer of protection between the vulnerable interior of the cell and the external environment. Cell walls can change and adjust their permeability, meaning how many particles they let into the interior of the cell (and when), as well as how many particles they let out (and when). This cell membrane somatization is incredibly useful for restoring the choice and power to *you*, in terms of what energy gets into your interior (and when) and what gets out (and when).

So, imagine there is a cell membrane surrounding you that has four settings:

1 In and Out: you welcome the energy coming in, and you let energy out as well.

2 Neither In nor Out: you do not let energy in, nor do you let energy out.

3 In but Not Out: you welcome energy in, but do not let any energy out.

4 Out but Not In: you let energy out, but do not welcome any in.

Now, pick a feeling or a quality of energy that you want to experiment with. For example, something like badass, energizing, loving, or sexy. Using that feeling or quality of energy, practice maneuvering between the four settings the next time you walk down the street, order coffee, or sit in a staff meeting. For example, practice letting sexy energy out, but not in. Or, practice letting loving energy in *and* out. Or, let energizing energy in, but not out. This practice is great for feeling centered and powerful even in the intense energies of the daily commute, fiery conversations, cocktail parties, management meetings, and everything in between.

THE DIAL

Right now, pay close attention to each of your five senses: what you can touch with the palms of your hands or surface of your body; a sound you can hear in the environment around you; a scent you can smell nearby, however faint; an image you see that draws your attention; and a taste lingering in your mouth—or one remembered.

With each of these five senses in turn, imagine there is a dial on each of the five, and dial it up. Let the sense fully in, thereby making it richer, fuller, more saturated, and more intense. For example, try touching one of your fingers to the palm of your hand and moving your finger slightly. Imagine there is a dial on the sensations you feel, both at the tip of your finger and on the palm of your hand. On a scale of one to ten, ten being the most intense, dial up the sensations you feel to about an eight or nine.

Relax any tension in your body that might be resisting feeling more. Let the sensations in fully, thereby making them richer, more saturated, and more intense. You can experiment with intentionally *leaning in* and thereby intensify the sensations by intentionally *reaching* toward them. And you can also experiment with intentionally *leaning out* and thereby intensify the sensations by attracting them toward you.

You will likely notice that either *leaning in* or *leaning out* works better for you. This is a great practice for everyday moments, as well as erotic ones where you want to intensify (or simplify) your sensual experience. The dial is also good for helping you turn an overwhelming moment into a calm one, or an ordinary moment into an ecstatic one.

The Feminine Genius skill of receiving requires your deliberate intention, consent, and action. Receiving is an important aspect of cultivating your light and letting your power flow. Like a radio antenna, receiving allows you to connect intimately with the divine field of Feminine Genius, your Oracle, and the people in your world. Receiving allows you to get nourished and juiced up, and to reap the rewards of all your hard work. Receiving lets you honor others for their tender hearts and their contributions. And receiving allows you to honor yourself as well, as you abstain from the collective dimming and refuse to diminish your gifts. Like a light bulb, receiving allows you to be seen as you truly are: a source of light.

How else can you let in—and let out—the truth of who you are?

If you wish for light, be ready to receive light.
RUMI

20

Un-Damming Your Power

Letting Your Voice Out
and Other Women In

At my age, in this still hierarchical time, people
often ask me if I'm "passing the torch." I explain
that I'm keeping my torch, thank you very much—
and I'm using it to light the torches of others.
GLORIA STEINEM

Woman, the spot upon which you now stand is golden.

You know how to transmit light through how you see and listen. You know how to excavate your deep desires. You are a devotee of your pleasure and presence, and can choose when, where, and how much to receive all the goodness that is quite surely aimed in your direction. Now it is time for you to bring your inner world out into this world. Now it is time to share yourself in a way that brings others closer, all without cramping your truth.

You and I have only a little more time together before you close this book and run off into the rest of your life. So that your power doesn't get stuck or stay stagnant, I want to highlight for you two areas that can potentially block your power and steal your life-force: how you express yourself and how you relate to other women.

To open your mouth and share with the world that which is asking to be lived *as* you and *through* you can be scary. You might fear that if you stand up, stick your neck out, say your piece, and ask for what you want, you might become a target, get shunned by your friends, or be abandoned by your beloveds. You might fear you will be pelted with rotten tomatoes, marked as high-maintenance, or labeled as crazy.

To open your heart and share with another woman the truth of who you are becoming can be even scarier. You might fear that other women are catty and competitive, not to be trusted. You might worry that you will get sized up, stabbed in the back, labeled as a loser, or left with a gut-twisting case of jealousy.

And yet. How else will things change unless you speak up about what you know needs to change? What you have to offer the world isn't crazy; it is needed to heal the world's own insanity. You don't have to stay locked in competition with other women; you can co-conspire to heal the war between us. In the quantum reality of interconnectivity, how else will you rise unless we all rise together?

By sharing your truth, you give others permission to do the same. By trusting other women to come close, you un-dam part of your power and let it flow. So before you set off to live the life of a Feminine Genius, let me give you all I can so you can let your voice out and let other women in.

LETTING YOUR VOICE OUT

> The most courageous act is still
> to think for yourself. Aloud.
> **COCO CHANEL**

I stood on red rocks, ankle deep in river water, wind in my hair. I was in Sedona, considered by many to be one of the most potent electromagnetic power spots on the globe, where the earth is the color of glowing embers. I was working with my longtime friend and public speaking coach, KC Baker, on a talk that I would soon give to several hundred women. So that I could embody the powerful and flowing qualities of water, and so that my words didn't get stuck or stagnant, she asked me to practice in the river.

KC's eyes shone with delight as she listened to me speak. When I faltered and paused, she waded into the river with me, sunlight catching the crystals hanging from her ears. She smiled and shared with me her KC-ism, as she has shared with countless women before me: "Don't say the right thing; say the true thing." I started again, trying to stay in my body while saying the truest things I know.

She listened, then rattled off a long, luxurious list of what was working about my talk, but a part of me still wondered if I was doing it all wrong, if my ideas were completely crazy, and if I would confuse or alienate my listeners. "The feelings and sensations of being anxious or nervous aren't a problem," KC reminded me. "The energy of those feelings and sensations is your power. You are feeling discomfort because your power is dammed up and can't quite get all the way through. Let's go eat lunch, and then let's try it again."

On that golden-lit afternoon, I was just one woman like any woman, trying to stay in my body and let my voice—and my power—run free. Literally and figuratively, no script to follow. Just feeling what I feel, knowing what I know, and simply saying what is true. In that Sedona river, I was just one woman like any woman, discovering again that perhaps as women we aren't *damned*, we are just dammed up.

It really takes something to open your mouth and share what is true, even to just one pair of ears. Georgia used to describe speaking up—at least outside of her work life—as something akin to dread on a good day, and something quite like terror on a bad one. A client of mine for several years, Georgia has always been sure-footed in her work as a project manager and consultant, confidently leading teams, meetings, and big-budget projects. But Georgia has carried through her whole life, and into her friendships and relationships, the restrictive belief that expressing what she wants to those she loves will at best inconvenience them, and at worse anger them and chase them away.

Georgia doesn't remember a time when her father didn't swing, without warning, from delightfully manic to despondent and depressed. Throughout her childhood, Georgia's father gave away her favorite toys, "borrowed" money she'd been given for birthdays and holidays, and, once, bought her a pony she didn't want and couldn't take care of because animals and hay made her physically sick. At one point, he suddenly moved out of the family home, and then several years later, moved back in, all without explanation. There is nothing quite like having your father, the god of your universe, make erratic decisions about your life. It can make you question what is true and wonder if speaking up is wise. It all led to Georgia concluding, "If I'm me, I won't be loved, and I won't belong."

Not everyone's past is as dramatic as Georgia's, but nearly every woman I know or have worked with has either a niggling—or raging—fear of letting her voice out, whether making a request or simply saying what is so. Because voicing your desires is a vulnerable and public declaration of what you care deeply about, you might tend to entomb your voice in the catacombs of your psyche. But when you detain your truths as your own noiseless little secrets, and when you squirrel away your wants over your lifetime, they dam your power. From my experience, expressing your desires—lovingly and powerfully, in a way that benefits both you and your listener—requires that you take not just one step, but four undaunted, un-damming steps.

Four Steps to Letting Your Voice Out

In the first step, you must embrace what it is that you desire. You must remember that it is okay—actually, more than okay—to simply love what you love, feel what you feel, know what you know, want what you want, and need what you need.

Now, you might believe, like Georgia did, that having needs—even the need to speak up about what you need—will make you seem needy or unlovable, and is therefore unacceptable. This is partly because you may have been, like Georgia was, groomed to be a "good girl," to be seen and not heard, and to please others before you please yourself (if you ever get around to pleasing yourself, that is). However, this first step requires you to strip off your Superwoman uniform, reach your hand down into the riverbed of your desires, and pull out a deep one, and then stand in your naked truth: in your body, connected innocently and intrepidly to what you love.

In the second step, you must positively presume that other people *want* to hear what you have to say. Other people are part of a Universe that, as pronoia proposes, is conspiring to shower you with blessings. So you must trust that other people aren't trying to block what you want and, in fact, might just have a lot of fun conspiring to help you get what you want. You must believe that what you desire may in fact be good for everyone, requiring in small or significant ways that everyone reach, grow, and expand to become who *they* are aching to become. This second step was the hardest for Georgia to wrap her head around, but in just a moment, I'll share how she benefited greatly from these positive presumptions.

In the third step of letting your voice out, you must, first and always, broadcast a field of appreciation, to yourself and to your listeners. Like you would first spread out a gemstone blanket, a soft surface upon which to place the gold nuggets you just pulled from the silt—and so that you and your listener can see the gems for what they are and can more easily admire the way they catch the light—it is extremely useful to likewise spread out an appreciative field before speaking up.

This step helps sift out of the conversation things like blame, shame, expectation, or proving yourself worthy, and helps whatever you share to land more cleanly with your listener. As you know, whatever type of field you choose will transmit through your body language, your energy, and the tone of your voice, as well as through the words you choose. In this third step, I suggest that you verbally share with your listeners something you appreciate about them, as a kind of stage-setting to sharing what you have to share. Even if your listeners don't—or can't—articulate what they feel, they will be positively affected by your appreciative field and your appreciative words.

In the fourth step, you must open up your mouth and let your voice out. To help you speak lovingly and powerfully, here's my recommendation. Start by asking this prompt, first of yourself, and then of your listener, "Know what I would love?"

Just like it is impossible to fake what truly brings you pleasure, it is impossible to fake what you love, what is true for you, and what is important to you. This prompt helps you to reposition your desire as something you adore, rather than something that might tarnish your value or lovability. And this prompt helps you express that desire to another, lovingly and powerfully. Here's how: When you ask yourself, "Know what I would love?" your Oracle pricks up her ears and starts to ponder, "Well, what *is* it that I would love?" Whatever question you pose to yourself, you will get some kinds of answers.

For example, if you ask yourself, "Know what I'm afraid of?" you will get a nice, long list of fears and doubts. If you ask yourself, "Know what is wrong with me?" you will get a nice, long list of your short-comings and crazies. In this case, when you ask yourself, "Know what I would love?" you will get a nice, long list of your desires: what you are devoted to, what you want, what you care about, what is important to you, and what is true for you.

Asking yourself this question is like panning for gold, when you plunge a tin pan into a riverbed; scoop up a bunch of water, rocks, and sand; then jiggle the contents around to see what gold will come to the surface. You dip your hand into the river water of your Oracle and pull out a gold nugget—a need, a request, a truth, a longing, or a deep desire to share with someone in your world.

What you find might be something you simply want witnessed or acknowledged, like a recent discovery about yourself, a vision you want to create, or a fresh idea that is dying to be heard. And what you find might be a proposal for something new or different, like a place to travel to, a course you'd like to take, a different way of parenting together, or an upgrade for a pattern of communication that is no longer working. You will know you have struck gold when you have fallen in love with the truth you have found, and can be its champion.

After asking this prompt to yourself, use it to start off a conversation wherein you share with your listener (or listeners) *what it is that you would love*. Instead of dipping you into disappointment or resentment, this prompt will help you more easily access your wells of joy, value, and love, and will therefore influence *what* you share and *how* you share it.

You can express the same desire with displeasure or delight. When you tap into what you love, the field you are emitting will feel distinct, your body language will look distinct, and your voice will sound distinct. Your listener will be more likely to hear you, receive you, and be interested in what you propose instead of having to armor against your critical or confusing field—and words.

Please do not misunderstand. I am not suggesting that you tidy and sanitize your desires before communicating them—a process that certainly could leave you even *more* tongue-tied. The truth that you pan for and find may indeed be messy. It does not have to be politically correct or easy for your listeners to hear. Just like KC reminded me back in that Sedona river, you needn't worry about sharing the "wrong" thing. Just share your truth.

The thing about your truth is that when you don't express it, it can make you some sort of sick. "Better out than in," my husband likes to say. He usually says this about mucous, vomit, or some purgative his body is using to get back to wellness. Gross, but true. When you shut your desires up inside you, even the fairly simple ones, they can become toxic. This is what started to happen for Georgia. About six months into our work together, she started dating Andrew, a man who was refreshingly reliable in contrast to her father, and to her past relationships. We got to work on Georgia's ability to speak up with Andrew, using the four steps I just outlined.

Georgia lived in the heart of the city, and Andrew lived in the suburbs with his two young boys, a ninety-minute drive away, near the boys' school and their mother. Between regular visits to Andrew and her work trips, Georgia was rarely home more than two days in a row. She was also having a flare up of an autoimmune disease she had wrestled with since her late teens. Her sleep, her eating, her yoga practice, and her inner equilibrium all began to slip.

The truth was that Georgia needed to stop traveling so much. She wanted to cozy up in her own home for even a week at a stretch, and just exhale. But in even thinking about bringing this up to Andrew, she nearly stopped breathing. She felt ungrateful, unaccommodating, and potentially unlovable.

"I felt a moment of wanting to resist and run away from the conversation for fear of finding out that what I wanted just wasn't possible, and then thought, 'aha, perhaps this is the very moment to lean in,'" Georgia reported to me after she had walked herself (and Andrew) through the four steps. "We had a really good conversation. And it was a very easy, uneventful conversation. Actually it was very eventful but only in the very best ways—I didn't die." She smiled. "And I actually felt heard and supported."

What you may not yet know, and what Georgia learned in her conversation—and in hundreds of subsequent conversations—is that the sound of a truth, expressed within a field of appreciation and without blame, shame, expectation, or proving yourself worthy, more often than not will perk up the inner ears of your listeners and call into being (and into action) a noble and resourceful part of them. Letting your listeners know what you value about them will let them know they need not brace for an attack but can instead open up to hear what you have to say. Expressed cleanly and powerfully, a deep desire will show its true face: a catalyst for goodness, growth, learning, and light—often for everyone involved.

In Georgia's inaugural conversation, for example, Andrew got to learn how to talk about things that he, too, used to sweep under the rug. He got to stretch into the kind of man he knew himself to be. Andrew's ex-wife got a clearer co-parent to coordinate with. Andrew and his kids got a more relaxed and healthy Georgia. Georgia got to exhale—and re-oxygenate herself with a more pleasurable, embodied, healthy daily life. And I got a client who no longer felt damned or dammed up.

As Georgia put it, "I felt, for possibly the first time in my romantic relationships, that what I want and need to be happy is important. My partner is curious about what that is and willing to be creative to make it happen." Expressing herself had always felt to Georgia as though she were in a tiny boat in a huge ocean without a paddle to help maneuver. She says, "Now the water is still vast, the storms still come, the waves still rock me, but now I have oars."

So as you let loose your truths and allow them to flow, here in the form of a practice are my four suggested steps for letting your voice out.

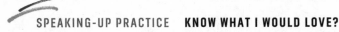

SPEAKING-UP PRACTICE   KNOW WHAT I WOULD LOVE?

Although you can apply this practice to speaking to larger groups, it is ideally suited to more intimate conversations with friends and partners.

1 First step, remind yourself of these positive presumptions about yourself and your desires:

- First of all, I really love my deep desires. I am a Genius for excavating them. I have an awesome Pandora's box.
- I have a direct line to the Divine, and I need to give the mic to my Oracle to share what is asking to be said *as* me and *through* me.
- I know that my needs are better out than in (and that they can fester when locked away inside). I can't wait to share these gems with my listeners and for these gems to be out in the light of day.
- I understand that no matter the response I receive, I am worthy, deserving of the best, and wholly lovable.
- I believe that my truth will likely change things for the better for myself as well as for my listeners, as is its nature.

2 Second step, remind yourself of these positive presumptions about your listeners.

- I presume that my listeners *want* very much to hear my truth.
- I assume that my listeners want me to have what I need and want, if not *help* me to get what I need and want.
- I assert that I can trust my listeners, and that it is safe to share with my listeners.

3 Third step, broadcast a field of appreciation, and lay it on thick to your listeners as well as yourself.

   (Heck, why not enjoy yourself and your listeners, as long as it is not wildly inappropriate for you to flirt so.)

I heartily suggest verbally sharing something you appreciate about your listeners as a positive preamble to your speaking up.

4   Fourth step, speak up! Start with the prompt, "Know what I would love?" and follow it with your request, need, want, truth, or deep desire.

As you ask the question of yourself and your listener, imagine speaking from your Oracle. Even just *thinking* of your Oracle while you are voicing the question will put a twinkle in your eye and intrigue in your voice.

For more formal situations, feel free to adjust your language. If you don't follow the letter of the law, you can still tap into the spirit of the law. For my client Astrid, who is a psychologist in the United States Navy, it isn't appropriate to start a meeting with her superior officer with, "Know what I would love?" But, connecting to what is important to her about the issue, and speaking up from there, is not only appropriate, it is vital to the powerful expression of her needs, as well as those of her patients and her workplace.

> When a woman tells the truth, she creates
> the possibility for more truth around her.
> **ADRIENNE RICH**

Can I give you insurance that this practice will work smoothly and effortlessly, every time? Truthfully, no. But to riff on a 12-step saying, I *can* promise that it works the more you work it. However, it is possible that even after all this, your listeners may still meet your expression with resistance, confusion, or suspicion. Your friend or partner may still say *no* to your request. This is not a failure or a disaster. Rather, just as you lifted the lid of the Pandora's box of a desire and inquired within (back in chapter 14), do the same with that *no* and get curious about their resistance, confusion, or suspicion. Dignify their hesitations, but explore them further.

As Georgia puts it, "What I'm learning about speaking my truth and asking for what I desire/want/need/long for is that their first response is not necessarily always (or often) their ultimate response. Or any real reflection on me. I'm noticing that there's often an initial reaction and then a subsequent response that represents some movement toward meeting the need/desire I'd expressed—not always in the way I envisioned, but sometimes even better. And just the movement toward meeting me and hearing me—and the willingness it represents—are meaningful to me." Even a *no* can help get you to a useful and truthful place.

In my experience, there is wisdom buried inside any *no*. Almost always, a set of important beliefs, fears, worries, and insights lies just underneath that *no*, and inquiring into your listener's concerns will not only reveal the wisdom there, but will also bring more intimacy, trust, and connection between you.

Georgia used to believe that her needs—like boundaries, sufficient sleep, and a spacious schedule—were self-indulgent luxuries for sissies who just couldn't take the heat. They were optional but certainly not essential. Now she sees them as markers of self-love, integrity, and grace. And she sees them as personal non-negotiables if she wants to show up in her life as the fullest version of herself. And Georgia no longer feels that what she has to say is crazy. She now knows that keeping it inside will make her feel insane.

I used to believe that just by opening my mouth I might confuse or repel, whether one listener or a thousand. Now I know, as you know, that there are really only two things you have control over: the quality of your awareness and to what you direct your awareness. You may not be able to control how a single person or a larger group will respond to what you share, but you can still appreciate them, enjoy yourself, wade into the river of your power, and let your voice come on out.

I now know, as you have come to know, that your voice is infused with the voice of the Sacred. That the stream of power that you sink into to find the nugget of your truth is the same stream of power that God herself uses to make the world go round. And that what you have to offer to the world is the answer to someone's prayer.

No, I am not having messianic delusions of grandeur. I am simply willing to tell the truth that you are—like we each are—an admittedly flawed, definitely enthusiastic, and always humble mouthpiece for Feminine Genius to have a word with the world. How else will new things come to be, if not through you? Your voice is yet one more way to let your power flow.

speaking up is golden
we can't wait to hear what you have to say

LETTING OTHER WOMEN IN

> Surround yourself only with people
> who are going to take you higher.
> **OPRAH WINFREY**

But, let's be honest. How easy is it to let comparison with—and mistrust of—another woman shut you down? Too easy, unfortunately.

Let me pause for a second and open the door to a dark, dusty closet, full of female skeletons, and beam the light of a flashlight inside. As you read the stories in this book, did you notice yourself shriveling as those women's stories loomed large? Did you feel jealous or judgmental? Did you say, "That might work for her, but not for poor old me?" As you get busy cultivating your light, you might pass through some shadow. The long and lethal competition between women is one of those dark underbellies indeed.

It is only fairly recently that a woman can make her own money, have a credit card in her own name, choose whether or not to marry or have children, and self-determine her life path. But for the thousands of years before now, if another woman was more desirable than you—via her beauty, family status, or dowry—she would get the house, husband, family, money, security, health, and esteem—and you could truly get nada. Your very life depended on men, and upon being better than other women in order to gain favor with men. To this day, the amount of energy a woman expends comparing herself to, shrinking around, and trying to beat out other women is astounding. And yet, if you cannot plug those energy leaks, you can never come into your own full power.

Fiercely feminist and a genius with the written word, Amelia is, in my opinion, the slightly Goth reincarnation of Gertrude Stein. Amelia joined my group mentorship program in order to come back home to her body, love her curves, and cultivate authentic friendships and relationships.

With a father who called her body "grotesque," and a mother who instilled crippling doubt in her skills, appetites, desires, and goals, Amelia got the message early on that everything she wanted was bad for her, and that she never achieved enough. She didn't trust her physical abilities or impulses one bit, and felt awkward, ugly, and ungainly. By age thirty-eight, when we met, her feelings of discomfort with herself—and her sense of being inferior to other women—had never left her.

Lacking encouraging role models among other women, Amelia assumed that what she did or thought might be attacked by those whose approval she wanted most. Her fear of herself and of others manifested as a phobia of falling. She lived in her head, and her body felt like a punishment. She closed herself up tight.

On our first weekend retreat, the group devised an experience for Amelia, where she was instructed into a "trust fall," falling backward into the waiting arms of ten other women. She nearly refused, not believing that the group could really hold her weight. But fall she did, and was caught fairly easily by ten pairs of arms. Being held up by a willing circle of sisters reverberated with meaning for Amelia, physically as well as metaphysically.

On our break, Amelia went down to a nearby river with a few of the other women from the retreat—women she might have seen as untouchable rivals in the past—to digest the profound shift that had happened for her. To her surprise, she climbed over the river rocks, the only time in her life where she felt sure-footed when crossing rough terrain. Her compatriots showered her with love and cheered her on. "Handholds and footholds opened up before my eyes. The world around me, my Mother Earth, caught me. I had new sisters to encourage me, and I felt strong," she explained to me later.

Amelia went on: "I feel now as though, literally and metaphorically, I will not fall. I feared being 'dropped,' abandoned, stepped over, and laughed at. Before, my body would have failed me. I would have been terrified, fallen, and hurt myself on those rocks. I feel now that because of these women, my goddess sisters, I can trust my deep 'feminine,' I can experience my body with joy instead of fear, and the world will catch me." Through the steadfast support of a group of novice Feminine Geniuses, Amelia got to experience her body as trustworthy and other women as trustworthy. This is also in store for you, when you want it.

Amelia was able to rewrite, as you will, too, her personal act 1 and a piece of our collective history of seeing other women as critics and adversaries. Amelia was able to see, as you will, too, that women who feel powerful in their own right (and who are not waiting for a culture to provide it or partner to prove it), need not compete with each other. You will see, as I have seen over fourteen beautiful years, that women who are at ease with their Oracles, at peace with Eros, and lit up with pleasure, become naturally generous and committed to everyone rising, together.

You can absolutely learn to see women as co-conspirators rather than the competition, each as yet another dazzling expression of the Feminine Divine rather than a threat to your livelihood, lovability, and value. When you let parts of yourself out, and let parts of them in, you un-dam your power.

Looked at it one way, the rivalry between women is kind of absurd. If I told you that a rose was turning green with envy of an orchid, you would probably think it ridiculous. "But, look," the rose would insist. "Just look at her plummy purple folds! She can subsist merely on mist alone. Orchids are so much more popular in bouquets these days. Roses are so passé. If I could only be more like an orchid."

"Silly rose," you'd reply. "Look at you. Really, look. You are gorgeous. Your scarlet whorls and delicate scent, your suit of velvet, studded with thorns . . . so mysterious! You are the symbol of the Divine Feminine, didn't you know? A rose, an orchid, a daisy; we need the variety like we need our next breath. The life-force that runs through the orchid runs through the rose; it animates all flowers, without exception." When you choose to see yourself and other women as the Divine Feminine sees every woman, every flowery face of the feminine must be revered, without exception.

My years of working with women have confirmed for me that, given a chance, a fellow Feminine Genius will not play power games with you but will delight in coaxing out your true power. She will not try to take you down a notch, but will get off by helping you burn brighter.

So then, it is vital that you consciously surround yourself with as many staggeringly magnificent women as possible, preferably all walking the path of Feminine Genius. You *want* to be bombarded by examples of self-expression, creativity, health, beauty, family, freedom, partnership, wifedom, business, activism, and friendship in ways you want for yourself as well. When you feel old, ugly, or unsuccessful, you *need* a sister to hold up a mirror and reflect your brightness. When your flame flickers, you *want* the torch held by a sister to help re-ignite your own.

Look, feeling jealous, judgmental, or small around other women is normal. It will happen. It might just happen *even more* as you surround yourself with other Feminine Geniuses. It's just that the questions you ask yourself must shift from, "Why is she so awesome, and I am so pathetic?" to "How can I get lit off her brilliance?" Here's a practice to help with that.

SISTERHOOD PRACTICE #1   GETTING LIT OFF ANOTHER WOMAN'S BRILLIANCE

This practice is to help you transform the crappy feelings you might experience when you're around other women. Instead of shrinking small or proving yourself as grand, this practice will direct you to get your torch re-lit from another woman's fire.

1 **Inquire:** What does your version of "She's so great, and I suck" or "I'm so great, and she sucks" feel like for you? Take note of your physical sensations and emotions, and try to identify what restrictive beliefs go with your feelings.

2 **Inquire further:** If these feelings and beliefs were inner truth-telling genies—daemons in demon's clothing—pointing out ways you are dimming your light, what is one way you can brighten?

3 **Inquire even further:** If these feelings and beliefs were signs to let you know "It is your turn to shine now," what would be your next step?"

I love this practice for the times when you find yourself surrounded by women who might intimidate you. But what about when you are nowhere near other women and are feeling isolated and alone? There is nothing quite like a band of other women to help you reconnect—to others, to yourself, and to the sacred. My prayer is that if you don't already have an existing group of like-minded sisters, you find one to join or start one of your own.

My first women's group lasted three years. It started as a book club with four other women, reading *Seductress: Women Who Ravished the World and Their Lost Art of Love,* by Betsy Prioleau. We circled up in each other's living rooms, to learn about women throughout history who experienced hot sex, epic adventure, wild successes, great careers, love and devotion, and fame and fortune, while defying all stereotypes of how a woman should look, behave, or think. The seductresses we read about weren't particularly good-looking, rich, or privileged by mainstream standards, but each was really workin' her unique brand of feminine strengths. We five stole liberally from the seductresses; we not only practiced strutting our stuff, but also learned to listen appreciatively, share vulnerably, be curious, coax out each other's visions, and see each other as beautiful and capable.

Another incarnation of a woman's group for me was a feminine version of a mastermind group, affectionately called a "mistressmind," in which eight women supported each other to employ our feminine values in our businesses and personal lives. Devotedly, for more than four years, we met over weekly phone calls and annual in-person retreats. We saw each other through big life events: companies bought and sold, pregnancies lost and babies' first steps, failed programs and windfalls, marriages, divorces, and happy singlehood.

Each word of encouragement or piercing insight I have received from women in groups like these takes into account the months and years we have spent together, practicing principles, sharing history, caring for each other, and getting lit off each other's brilliance. In every in-person program I create, I always group up the participants so they can begin to taste this for themselves, and so they can carry the women's group format into their lives long after we've worked together. (For forming a women's group yourself, and for forming a book club based on this book, you can find my guidelines at liyanasilver.com/bookresources.)

And if something formalized like a women's group, mistressmind, or book club isn't your thing, or isn't your thing *today*, you can still start creating a tribe of like-minded sisters simply by having one brave conversation at a time, with one woman at a time. Goddess knows where it will lead you. As Pam, a reader of mine on Facebook puts it, "Whenever one of us shares, and is brave enough to be vulnerable, it gives all of us permission to be just a little bit more so. And that is a treasure."

You already know how to do it. But to help you dust off your skills, here's a review.

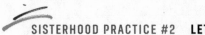

SISTERHOOD PRACTICE #2   LETTING ANOTHER WOMAN IN

When you reach for an hors d'oeuvre on the same tray, sit next to each other on a playground bench, rub elbows around the water cooler at work, or ride-share after a play—for complete strangers and friends you want to know better—here's one way to open the door of your heart, connect to a sister, and do your part to dismantle the barriers that have existed for too long between women. Here's how you help another woman to re-light her torch off your own.

1   Broadcast a field of appreciation.

2   Start by telling this woman something you appreciate about her. Enjoy yourself while you enjoy this other woman.

3   Connect to your Oracle and pan for gold. Open your kimono a bit. Let your voice come out.

    Tell her about the ways you have been seeing that you aren't crazy—it is the world that is nuts.

    Ask her what she deeply desires and share your own. Ask her about what it feels like for her when her power is dammed up, and what it feels like for her when her power is flowing. Ask her when she has felt most present. Ask her if she is squirmy or sure-footed when it comes to receiving. Ask what she knows about navigating the dark. Ask how she is doing with cultivating her light.

    Don't worry about saying or asking the wrong thing, just say what is true for you and ask what's true for her.

4   Listen to her. Continue to enjoy yourself while enjoying this other woman. Let this other women in.

5   Watch what blooms in the rare and hallowed space between you. And notice that things start to look that much brighter.

There are two ways of spreading light:
to be the candle or the mirror that reflects it.
EDITH WHARTON, "Vesalius in Zante"

And yet, the questions may still linger, such as: "Can I really bring my whole self, my true self, my Feminine Genius self to my life? Won't I bowl people over? Won't I be asking too much of them? Won't I be too much to take? Won't they reject and skewer me? If I let loose my voice, will everyone leave? If I offer myself to the world, will anyone care?"

I have supported women countless times as they decided to leave five-year, fourteen-year, and thirty-year partnerships, and as some of their longtime friendships fell away painfully. And I have likewise supported women as they attracted startlingly synchronistic new friendships, re-devoted themselves to breathing life into their long-term relationships, or realized they actually prefer being single. Feminine Genius is just as likely to urge you to stay, as she is to let you know it's time to go.

Regardless, 100 percent of the time, each woman who has stopped being someone she is not, and who has started being just who she is, has eventually become a beacon for what I call "right-fitting" friendships and intimate relationships. Each woman who has offered herself fully to the world has found that there is room for more than one powerful woman. In fact, what is needed most is a world full of Feminine Geniuses.

The mistrust between women is timeless, but step-by-step you can transmute competition into collaboration, jealousy into trust, isolation into friendship, and disconnection into an intimate tribe or larger network. You will rise or fall to the company you keep, so it becomes requisite to keep yourself in the company of great women, relating as sisters, keeping each other aflame. Every time you open your heart and your mouth, it sets another woman free to do the same.

I want you to fully embrace the awesome reality that when it comes to living as a Feminine Genius—whether you prefer to lie low or are out there in the public eye—you are becoming a leader and an icon of sorts. You are becoming an agent for change, whether you start with a single friend or your larger community. You are becoming a rare and miraculous sight: a woman who speaks her truth, a brightly burning torch upon which other women can get themselves lit, a woman who will light, lead, and heal our world.

Sister, as we start to come to a close, notice this: you have long since crossed a line in the sand. On that side, fitting in and following the script were your gods. On this side, you are also God, guided by the jubilant and intrepid voice of your Oracle. Coming home to yourself must come first; whom you choose to make home with comes after.

You have long since crossed the line, dear heart, and once you have un-dammed your power and tasted your truth, there is no going back. Your like-kind and the world as you envision it can't wait to meet you here.

and we are so, so glad you are here

of the storm of all that you feel. You let the Queen of the Dark burn away that which you no longer need.

You hold the fiery mystery of the stars in your bones, and you shine like a searchlight. You know that all parts of you, working together as a unified whole, is the mark of Genius. You have all you need within you to navigate the dark night and walk proudly into your bright life.

You Remembered to Take Your Body with You You have welcomed your prodigal girl child, at once innocent and divine.

You know there is no spot on which God is not, no place that is not holy—including every inch of your flesh. You have discovered an Oracle between your thighs, learned to speak her native tongue, and let her help you steer your whole life.

You have unearthed your deep desires as a zip-line to the Feminine Divine.

Emboldened and empowered, venerated and integrated, you know how to use erotic energy as fiery fuel to strengthen your body so you can bring through your passion. You can allow Eros to ally you with pleasure, which will ally you with confidence. You can allow Eros to bind you to the Sacred, bringing meaning into your everyday life.

You have cultivated your inner world. You have fortified the connection between your inner world and the other world. You now see the Beloved's face in the looking glass. Well remembered!

You Have Turned Your Light On Woman. You. Have. Turned. Yourself. On. And the secret under your smile says that you know how you help keep the candle flame lit.

Because: The more pleasure, the more truth. The more presence, the more power. The more life-force, the more light.

You now know that what you appreciate, appreciates. Your looking and listening can influence how anyone speaks, thinks, feels, and acts—yourself included. And when in doubt, you can flirt, dance, and pleasure yourself back to life.

You are now in dialogue with all of Creation, and Creation is so glad you are here. Get ready to drink in this shower of blessings; sweet, funky, and fierce as they may be. Oh, you don't have to take everything

21

Bringing Your Feminine Genius To Life
Coming Home and Becoming Home

One is not born, but rather becomes, a woman.
SIMONE DE BEAUVOIR, *The Second Sex*

During a vacation in Mexico a few years ago, I walked along the beach back to my rented villa after meeting friends for dinner. Fish tacos and good conversation had distracted me from noticing that night had fallen quickly, and I could barely see my bare feet on the sand as I headed toward home. Ahead in the dusk, I suddenly saw an otherworldly, glowing light that lifted into the air and headed out toward the open sea.

A little nervous, because I wondered if what I was seeing was an odd drone or an alien spacecraft, I came upon a group of women and girls in a circle around a bonfire, talking and giggling in hushed voices. I couldn't tell what they were saying, but it felt private, sacred, and celebratory. I imagined a cauldron between them, their cheeks lit by the glowing coals and the exchange of secrets.

I got close enough to see that each woman held a white paper lantern, its walls as thin as moth wings. One by one, each woman lit the candle inside her lantern. One by one, each woman held her glowing globe high. And one by one, each lantern, made buoyant by the heat inside, lifted out of the hands of these women, caught the evening wind, and floated out toward the horizon. I watched as the little fires flickered and did not burn out, but rose higher, regally shining through the luscious night, proudly laying a path of light.

Like these little Mexican fire lanterns, dear one, you too have gotten lit, held yourself aloft, hitched a ride on the wind, and are now about to sail out over the ocean of the rest of your life.

When you picked up this book, you may have felt numb, pissed off, and tired—fated to a dim future. Yet as you have read and practiced, you have confirmed your destiny as a living, breathing miracle. Your life is your own. You are a benediction. And a temple.

You have set down self-flagellation and self-deprecation, because you know they can't carry you to where you are going. Where once you felt riddled with holes, you have filled those holes with wholeness. Befitting your holiness, you have learned to capitalize the word *Woman*. Sitting as still as you wish or grinding your hips, you embody divine light. Where you once felt too much or not nearly enough, now you know you are just right. Since you know that *you* are what the Goddess looks like, you can invite us all to *enjoy the view*.

These are miracles

your miracles

drink them like honey

Whether you choose to walk swiftly or slowly, to make good time or take your sweet time, this path is now yours.

This provocative ride is over, and now *you* begin.

Wild applause! Standing ovation! Confetti! You did it! We're done!

And yet. As the alchemical dictum declares, "In my ending is my beginning." So as we celebrate *our* ending and all that *you* are beginning, let us be clear: your Feminine Genius path has just begun.

And really, it never ends.

Woman

you are always coming home

as well as becoming Home

You have come far and you have come wide. You have learned and y[ou] have unlearned. You have died and been reborn. Let's get the step-[by-]step highlights from this Heroine's Journey we have taken together.

You Went Straight for the Source   You loosened your grip on the script a[nd] found your own way. You found yourself far from crazy—you fou[nd] yourself brave and beautiful. You denounced people pleasing and [the] prison of pretty, and instead chose wisdom. You stopped the war w[ith] yourself, and realized that the only thing you lost was your desir[e to] do battle.

You gave up being perfect—as in flawless, finished, and invu[lner]able—and you see yourself instead as wondrously and perfectly m[ade]. The jar with the cracks needn't be tossed on the trash heap; it is [won]drously and perfectly made for watering the garden.

You know that walking the path of the Feminine Genius i[s the] highest-stakes, highest-reward game in town. And you're in good [with] the headmistress of learning and growing, so you've got a lif[etime] supply of gold stars.

Because the conversation with the Divine happens right here[and] now, and is not limited to ashrams, synagogues, yoga mats, or [medi]tation cushions, you know that every moment is communion[. And] there is nowhere you could go, and nothing you could do, to fal[l from] the web of the All That Is.

You Birthed Your Light in Your Dark   You reached into the other wo[rld,] brought back treasures. You learned that going up and down, an[d a]round and round, is simply your nature. You found yourself at [home]

in. You know how to deliberately wield your light with care and skill. Invisible is just as good a choice as full-wattage. What you receive is your choice.

Take it further. Bless us with your ecstasy. Lead with your intuitive intelligence. Commune with your truth, and tell us loud and clear what you hear. Let other women catch you, and let them catch you on fire.

your light is a blessing and a prayer,
as potent as fire,
as necessary as air

So now what? Claim your triumphs. Drink your miracles like honey. Boldly embody your Genius. Throw back your head and profess your joy. Exalt. Woman, you have arrived.

And remember, right after an arrival is yet another departure. You are never static. What Woman can stay still for long? Soon, Feminine Genius will be pouring through you, aching anew.

You are always moving, retreating, expanding, bending, breaking, mending. You are always falling and then again rising. Rising through the sky at night, a holy, holy sphere of light.

You are always coming home, and you are always becoming Home.

you are always
becoming
Woman

Thank You

If the only prayer you ever say in your
entire life is "thank you," that would suffice.

MEISTER ECKHART

Nathan, for being the loam from which I bloom, for valiantly holding down the fort while I let loose my roar. When we lose our way, we always find it together.

Mom, for making me. And for seeing me like the Divine sees us all: precious, a wonder; utterly and joyously loved. Dad, for always looking beyond the veil. And for your absolute, unabashed, infectious love of life. Kathryn, for sweet, strong sisterhood, literally and literarily. Erika, sistah, for being my first idol.

My clients, WEE women, Man Whisperers, and Feminine Badasses, for taking the path less traveled, and for the honor of helping to rewrite your story in splendor.

Kate, for making art out of it all. For meeting me in the heart of the dark. For staying. Anika, for no-bullshit, all-star friendship from the Rio Grande to the stream. Sera, for setting me up on my first blind date with the Divine Feminine. For helping me feel the difference between truth and untruth.

KC, the manifestingest motha, for reminding me that who we are is love. Wendy, for seeing beauty wherever you look, including at me. And for gorgeous photos, always. Alisa, for cycling with me in unending friendship. Alexandra, for making dances that imitate life and for being my BFF. My soul brother, Bryan, for making art out of love.

Regena Thomashauer, for standing for me, for standing for pussies everywhere. Carla Camou, for teaching me how to not die from emotions. Michelle Masters, Deb Kern, Carl Buchheit, for mentorship of the highest order. For teaching me that being human is not a fallen condition. Kassy Shekeloff, Ilana Firestone, the Morehouse community, and Dr. Patricia Taylor, for expanding my definition of pleasure.

The Seductress Salon and women of the Mistressmind, for growing the Goddess in me. Annie, for demanding that I howl, for suggesting that I self-regulate. Nisha, for making and breaking the mold of "sistering." Jena, for paving the way, and modeling self-celebration. Stacey, for championing my voice, even beyond the point of no return. Jennifer, for holding me strong when I was going down.

Sabrina, for gracefully embodying the fierce feminine. Domenica, for showing me the dark is delicious. Lisa, for sassy, sexy, Shakti sisterhood, even when I whine. Saida and Sol, for sexy integrity and succulent friendship. Lexie, for mad grass and magic. Susan, for your womancave, weekly composting sessions, and *perfect* design. Jessie, for rock star support. Mary, for the Fig.

Michael Ellsberg, for your ballsy views, and for being my word angel. Ibrahim, for removing degrees of separation. Alia, for feminine medicine. Eleanor, for helping me "burn in the fire of my own medicine." Sonya, for personifying sweet ferocity. Kim, for modeling gentle bitchery. Julia, for your nerve—and verve. And films of beauty, always.

Gangaji, for kindly reminding me that all sickness is homesickness. Dolano, for pointing the way to waking the fuck up.

Chantal Pierat, for encouraging me. Laura Yorke, for taking me on. Jennifer Brown, for acquiring me. Haven Iverson, for orchestrating me. Joelle Hann, for editing me. All of team Sounds True, you mystical band of upstarts—including Leslie, Lindsey, Christine, and Kira—for helping me facet a diamond out of a hard hunk of rock.

Notes

CHAPTER 1

1   Jennifer Siebel Newsom (director). *Miss Representation*, 2001, therepresentationproject.org/film/miss-representation/.

2   Margaret Renkl, "The Scary Trend of Tweens with Anorexia," *CNN Online*, August 2011, cnn.com/2011/HEALTH/08/08/tweens.anorexia.parenting/.

3   Chris Iliades, MD, "Stats and Facts about Depression in America," *Everyday Health*, January 2013, everydayhealth.com/hs/major-depression/depression-statistics/.

4   Katherine Bindley, "Women and Prescription Drugs: One in Four Takes Mental Health Meds," *Huffington Post*, August 2011, huffingtonpost.com/2011/11/16/women-and-prescription-drug-use_n_1098023.html.

5   Cynthia R. Bulik, PhD, "Survey Finds Disordered Eating Behaviors among Three out of Four American Women," University of North Carolina at Chapel Hill School of Medicine, April 2008, med.unc.edu/www/newsarchive/2008/april/survey-finds-disordered-eating-behaviors-among-three-out-of-four-american-women.

6   Shaun Dreisbach, "Shocking Body-Image News: 97% of Women Will Be Cruel to Their Bodies Today," *Glamour Magazine Online*, February 2011, glamour.com/story/shocking-body-image-news-97-percent-of-women-will-be-cruel-to-their-bodies-today.

7   Madison Park, "WHO: 1 in 3 Women Experience Physical or Sexual Violence," *CNN Online*, June 20, 2013, cnn.com/2013/06/20/health/global-violence-women/.

8   National Sexual Violence Resource Center, "Statistics about Sexual Violence," 2012, 2013, 2015, nsvrc.org/sites/default/files/publications_nsvrc_factsheet_media-packet_statistics-about-sexual-violence_0.pdf.

9   Ibid.

10 Sandra McKay and Nancy H. Hornberger, *Sociolinguistics and Language Teaching* (Cambridge, UK: Cambridge University Press, 1995), 226.

11 International Labour Organization, "Forced Labour, Modern Slavery, and Human Trafficking," International Labour Organization online (1996–2016), ilo.org/global/topics/forced-labour/lang--en/index.htm.

12 Maeve Duggan, "Online Harassment," Pew Research Center, October 2014, pewinternet.org/2014/10/22/online-harassment/.

CHAPTER 2

1 Mirabai Starr, *Saint Teresa of Avila: Passionate Mystic* (Boulder, CO: Sounds True, 2007), 65.

CHAPTER 4

1 Bob Samples, *The Metaphoric Mind: A Celebration of Creative Consciousness* (Reading, MA: Addison-Wesley, 1976), 26.

CHAPTER 6

1 Alisa Vitti, HHC, *WomanCode: Perfect Your Cycle, Amplify Your Fertility, Supercharge Your Sex Drive, and Become a Power Source* (New York: HarperOne, 2013), 6.

CHAPTER 7

1 Karla McLaren, *The Language of Emotions: What Your Feelings Are Trying to Tell You* (Boulder, CO: Sounds True, 2010), 31.

CHAPTER 8

1 Mirabai Starr, *Caravan of No Despair: A Memoir of Loss and Transformation* (Boulder, CO: Sounds True, 2016), xiii.

2 Mirabai Starr, *Saint Teresa of Avila*, 80.

CHAPTER 10

1 Riane Eisler, *Sacred Pleasure: Sex, Myth, and the Politics of the Body—New Paths to Power and Love* (New York: HarperCollins, 1996), 145.

2 Marilyn Frye, *Willful Virgin: Essays in Feminism* (Freedom, CA: Crossing Press, 1992), 133.

CHAPTER 11

1 Naomi Wolf, *Vagina: A New Biography* (New York: HarperCollins, 2012), 240.

2 Eisler, *Sacred Pleasure*, 60.

3 Ibid., 59.

4 Ibid., 49.

5 Ibid., 373.

CHAPTER 12

1 Wolf, *Vagina*, 4.

CHAPTER 14

1 Rupert Sheldrake, "Morphic Resonance and Morphic Fields—An Introduction," sheldrake.org/research/morphic-resonance/introduction.

2 Rupert Sheldrake, "Morphic Resonance," sheldrake.org/research/morphic-resonance.

CHAPTER 15

1 Caroline Myss, *Advanced Energy Anatomy: The Science of Co-Creation and Your Power of Choice* (Boulder: Sounds True, 2002), audio book.

2 Eve Ensler, *The Vagina Monologues* (New York: Villard Books, 1998), xx.

CHAPTER 16

1 Wikipedia, "Heresy," last modified December 12, 2016, en.wikipedia.org/wiki/Heresy#cite_note-4.

SPECIAL THANKS TO OVERTHEMOONMAG.COM WHO PUBLISHED MY ARTICLE IN 2015 WITH CONTENT SIMILAR TO THE CHAPTER "SEX RE-EDUCATION."

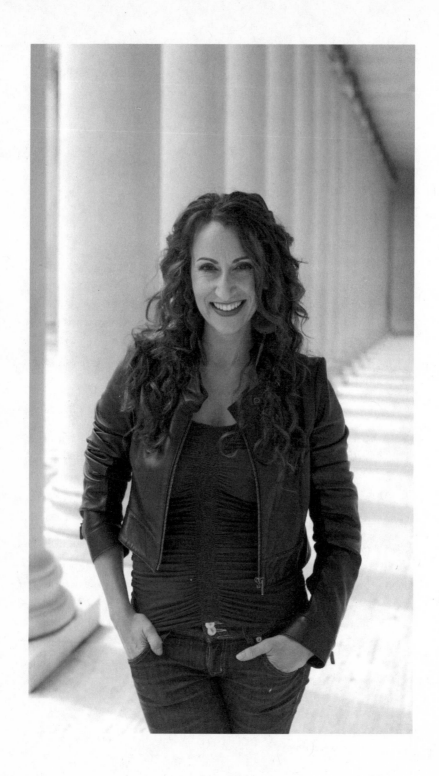

About The Author

iYana Silver is a torch-holder for the world-to-be in which the epidemic of women self-haters has long become absurd. For over fourteen years she has been coaching, mentoring, writing, speaking, leading live retreats and digital programs, supporting woman after woman to become simply and fully herself.

"Someone finally gets me!" is what most people say when they cross paths with LiYana, whether they are (as they have been) edge-cutting entrepreneurs, corporate professionals, artists, healers, social activists, mothers returning to work or balancing career with family, Fortune 500 leaders, or even a shaman or two.

LiYana works immersively with women in her six-month mentorship program, The Embodiment Experience, as well as in private sessions. She connects closely with women in the virtual sphere via her signature course, Ignite Your Feminine Genius, and her Facebook community. LiYana is a Holistic Health Coach, certified by the American Association of Drugless Practitioners, and holds a master's certification in Transformational NLP. Her eyebrow-raising work has been featured in the *Huffington Post*, *Forbes*, *Jezebel*, and Emerging Women.

LiYana was born to new-age, free-thinking parents, raised on an intentional community in northern New Mexico, and grew up with garden veggies and hand-me-downs. (She has yet to get back in the box.) Nowadays, when she's not caressing her computer keyboard, she's dancing, being a silly, enchanted mama, falling in love with her husband all over again, tending her close friendships, smelling the fresh herbs growing on her windowsill, or painting in oils.

Some shoulders on which LiYana gratefully stands and which have greatly inspired her life and work: Carl Buchheit, Carla Camou, and Michelle Masters of Transformational NLP at NLP Marin, Integrative Nutrition, Vipassana mindfulness meditation, Vedic Tantra, Hatha

Vinyasa Yoga, Anthony Robbins, Landmark Education, Osho, Dolano, Gangaji, the Family Systems work of Bert Hellinger, and the thought-leadership of David Deida, Ilana Firestone and Kassy Sheklehoff (and all the teachers) at Morehouse, Alison Armstrong of PAX, Regena Thomashauer of Mama Gena's School of Womanly Arts, Sabrina Chaw, Riane Eisler, Dr. Christiane Northrup, Dr. Patricia Taylor of Expanded Orgasm, Alexandra Beller Dances, Jodi White of Dance Theatre Seven, and her own extraordinary parents, Roland Silver and Beverly Pollack-Silver.

LiYana makes home with her husband and son, and can be found at LiYanaSilver.com.

About Sounds True

Sounds True is a multimedia publisher whose mission is to inspire and support personal transformation and spiritual awakening. Founded in 1985 and located in Boulder, Colorado, we work with many of the leading spiritual teachers, thinkers, healers, and visionary artists of our time. We strive with every title to preserve the essential "living wisdom" of the author or artist. It is our goal to create products that not only provide information to a reader or listener, but that also embody the quality of a wisdom transmission.

For those seeking genuine transformation, Sounds True is your trusted partner. At SoundsTrue.com you will find a wealth of free resources to support your journey, including exclusive weekly audio interviews, free downloads, interactive learning tools, and other special savings on all our titles.

To learn more, please visit SoundsTrue.com/freegifts or call us toll-free at 800.333.9185.

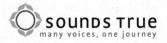

SOUNDS TRUE
many voices, one journey